Adolescent Counseling

Adolescent Counseling

Second Edition

Editors

MKC Nair
DSc PhD MD MMedSc (Australia) MBA MA
Director
NIMS Spectrum Child Development Research Centre
Thiruvananthapuram, Kerala, India
Former Vice Chancellor, Kerala University of Health Sciences
Founder Director, Child Development Centre, Thiruvananthapuram

Preeti M Galagali
MD (Ped) PGD AP (Adolescent Pediatrics) FIAP
Director
Bengaluru Adolescent Care and Counseling Centre
Clinical Lead, Adolescent Health Services
Department of Pediatrics and Adolescent Medicine
Manipal Hospital
Bengaluru, Karnataka, India

Foreword

Paul Swamidhas Sudhakar Russell

JAYPEE

JAYPEE BROTHERS MEDICAL PUBLISHERS
The Health Sciences Publisher
New Delhi | London

Jaypee Brothers Medical Publishers (P) Ltd

Headquarters
EMCA House, 23/23-B
Ansari Road, Daryaganj
New Delhi 110 002, India
Landline: +91-11-23272143, +91-11-23272703
+91-11-23282021, +91-11-23245672
e-mail: jaypee@jaypeebrothers.com

Corporate Office
4838/24, Ansari Road, Daryaganj
New Delhi 110 002, India
Phone: +91-11-43574357
Fax: +91-11-43574314
e-mail: jaypee@jaypeebrothers.com

Overseas Office
JP Medical Ltd.
83, Victoria Street, London
SW1H 0HW (UK)
Phone: +44-20 3170 8910
e-mail: info@jpmedpub.com

EU GPSR Authorised Representative
Logos Europe, 9 rue Nicolas Poussin
17000, La Rochelle, France
Phone: +33 (0) 6 67 93 73 78
e-mail: contact@logoseurope.eu

Website: www.jaypeebrothers.com
Website: www.jaypeedigital.com

Inquiries for bulk sales may be solicited at: jaypee@jaypeebrothers.com

Adolescent Counseling

First Edition: 2016
Second Edition: **2025**

ISBN: 978-93-5696-584-3

Printed at Officenow India

Dedication to

Over one lakh children, adolescents and their parents who have helped us to make counseling a passion in life

Contributors

Anil Kumar TV
Professor and Head
Department of Psychiatry
Government Medical College
Ernakulam, Kerala, India

Anuradha HS
Director, Tots2 Teens Health Care
Founder Confident Parenting Hub
Pediatrics
Gunasheela Maternity
and IVF Center
Bengaluru, Karnataka, India

Babu George
Formerly Director, CDC Kerala and
Developmental Pediatrician
KIMS Health
Thiruvananthapuram, Kerala, India

Chitra Dinakar
Professor and Head
Department of Pediatrics
St Martha's Hospital
Bengaluru, Karnataka, India

Fr MK George SJ
General Counsellor
Superior General of the Society
of Jesus, Rome

Harikumar SK
Physician and Director
SK Consultancy
Thiruvananthapuram, Kerala, India

Indira MS
Consultant Child Psychologist
Child Development Centre
Medical College Campus
Thiruvananthapuram, Kerala, India

Indu PS
Professor and Head
Department of Community
Medicine
Government Medical College
Kollam, Kerala, India

Leena Sumaraj
Senior Research Coordinator
Child Development Centre
Medical College Campus
Thiruvananthapuram, Kerala, India

Manoj Kumar Sharma
Professor of Clinical Psychology
Consultant and Head, SHUT
(Service for Healthy Use of
Technology) Clinic
Department of Clinical Psychology
National Institute of Mental Health
and Neuro Sciences (NIMHANS)
Bengaluru, Karnataka, India

Mercy Sebastian
Assistant Professor of Clinical
Psychology
Department of Psychiatry
Government Medical College
Thiruvananthapuram, Kerala, India

Mini K Paul
Consultant Psychologist
Child Development Centre
Medical College Campus
Thiruvananthapuram, Kerala, India

MKC Nair
Director
NIMS Spectrum Child
Development Research Centre
Thiruvananthapuram, Kerala, India
Former Vice Chancellor, Kerala
University of Health Sciences
Founder Director, Child
Development Centre,
Thiruvananthapuram

Narendra Nath Samantaray
Assistant Professor
Department of Clinical Psychology
National Institute of Mental Health
and Neuro Sciences (NIMHANS)
Bengaluru, Karnataka, India

Neema Sitapara
Consultant Pediatrician and
Adolescent Counselor
Department of Pediatrics
Maa Sharda Child Care Hospital
Rajkot, Gujarat, India

Neha John
Junior Consultant
SHUT (Service for Healthy use of
Technology) Clinic
Department of Clinical Psychology
National Institute of Mental Health
and Neuro Sciences (NIMHANS)
Bengaluru, Karnataka, India

Newton Luiz
Consultant Pediatrician
Department of Pediatrics
Dhanya Mission Hospital
Thrissur, Kerala, India

Nitin Anand
Additional Professor of Clinical
Psychology
Consultant, SHUT (Service for
Healthy use of Technology) Clinic
Department of Clinical Psychology
National Institute of Mental Health
and Neuro Sciences (NIMHANS)
Bengaluru, Karnataka, India

Paul Swamidhas Sudhakar Russell
Senior Professor
Child and Adolescent Psychiatry Unit
Christian Medical College
Vellore, Tamil Nadu, India

Preeti M Galagali
Director
Bengaluru Adolescent Care
and Counseling Centre
Clinical Lead, Adolescent
Health Services
Department of Pediatrics
and Adolescent Medicine
Manipal Hospital
Bengaluru, Karnataka, India

Raghavendra Kumar K
Founder Director
Mana Mandira Healthcare
Consultant Child and Adolescent
Psychiatrist
Honorary Consultant, Indira Gandhi
Institute of Child Health (IGICH)
Bengaluru, Karnataka, India

Rajesh Kumar
Assistant Professor of
Clinical Psychology
Department of Clinical Psychology
National Institute of Mental Health
and Neuro Sciences (NIMHANS)
Bengaluru, Karnataka, India

Rekha RS
Formerly Preschool Consultant
Child Development Centre
Medical College Campus
Thiruvananthapuram, Kerala, India

Resmi VR
Developmental Therapist
Child Development Centre
Medical College Campus
Thiruvananthapuram, Kerala, India

Rev TJ Thomas
Former Director
Thomas Mar Athanasius Institute
of Counselling Centre
Kottayam, Kerala, India

Shubhada Khirwadkar
Consultant Pediatrician
and Psychologist
Project Director, Community based
Interventions for Management
and Prevention of Malnutrition in
Children and Adolescents in Tribal
Area of Melghat
Counseling Psychologist
MAHAN Trust's Tribal Hospital
Amravati, Maharashtra, India

Shweta Sunil
Research Scholar
Department of Clinical Psychology
SHUT Clinic (Service for
Healthy Use of Technology)
National Institute of Mental Health
and Neuro Sciences (NIMHANS)
Bengaluru, Karnataka, India

Sonny Jose
Professor and Director
International Relations and Mobility
Loyola College of Social Sciences
Thiruvananthapuram, Kerala, India

Sreyoshi Ghosh
Consultant Child and Adolescent
Psychiatrist and Psychotherapist
Cadabams Hospitals
Bengaluru, Karnataka, India

Sukanya Ray
Assistant Professor
School of Human Ecology
Tata Institute of Social Sciences
Mumbai, Maharashtra, India

Suresh Kumar G
Former Registrar, CDC, Kerala
Chairperson, FPAI Kerala Chapter
Thiruvananthapuram, Kerala, India

Susha Janardanan
Director and Chief Mentor
Bright Ray Training, Research
Consulting Services
(A Centre for Mental Health and
Well-being)
Thiruvananthapuram, Kerala, India

Swati Ghate
Joint Director
Babylon's Newton Institute of Child and Adolescent Development
Jaipur, Rajasthan, India

Vidhu Kumar
Professor and Head
Department of Psychiatry
Government TD Medical College
Alappuzha, Kerala India

Vinayak Koparde
Associate Professor
Department of Child and Adolescent Psychiatry
Jawaharlal Nehru Medical College
Belagavi, Karnataka, India

Foreword

There is no ambiguity about the medical and psychological vulnerability of adolescents. The emotional and intellectual functioning of adolescents is forever changing along with their physiological changes interacting with their environmental demands. This period of a person, despite their innate difficulties, is one of the most important preparatory stages for efficient adulthood. Unfortunately, for many, these normative and added problems become stressful to compromise in their developmental course.

Counseling can be useful for adolescents to improve their existing internal and external resources or can help undo their compromised developmental-emotional-intellectual trajectory. The hundreds of different counseling techniques available today can be effectively used at different levels of the caregiving pathways. They can vary from simple, brief, supportive methods at primary-care settings to complicated, lengthy, multi-model techniques that are offered in specialized settings.

Adolescent Counseling focuses on the former type of counseling where easy-to-use techniques for day-to-day hassles faced by the adolescents are addressed. The initial chapters of this easy-to-carry around paperback have been compiled to introduce the readers to the developing cognitive process of adolescents and the essential tenets that form the basis for counseling. The later chapters have discussed specific concerns associated with this at- risk group. I trust this book will help all those in the primary-care sector to effectively hold hands with the adolescents until further counseling referrals can be organized.

Paul Swamidhas Sudhakar Russell
Professor
Child and Adolescent Psychiatry Unit
Christian Medical College
Vellore, Tamil Nadu, India

Preface to the Second Edition

Adolescents aged 10–19 years constitute 18% of the Indian population. They are our demographic dividend, and their well-being will determine the health and progress of India. There has been a surge in mental disorders in the post covid era amongst adolescents and adults. The global catastrophic events like wars, terrorism, climate change, natural disasters and food insecurity have added to the mental distress. Digital technology advances, artificial intelligence and social media algorithms have altered the social milieu in which adolescents grow. The rise in individualism, the need for immediate gratification, westernization and globalization has increased the emotional turmoil in society on the whole. Failure to understand and manage these new age issues has led to increased conflicts between adolescents and their caregivers and educators. Effective counseling can help adolescents, parents and teachers to cope with these emerging challenges.

Adolescence is an age of opportunity, rapid biopsychosocial growth and development, high energy, and creativity, where the foundations of health are strengthened. This is also the period where the effects of adversities faced earlier in life can be diminished. A healthy lifestyle adopted in adolescence usually tracks into adulthood and over generations. Emotional lability, reward seeking behavior, identity crisis, curiosity, negative peer pressure and experimentation with risk behavior can alter the developmental trajectory leading to poor health consequences. Counseling in adolescence promotes physical, mental, emotional, and social well-being. It also gives adolescents a safe space to discuss their problems and adopt healthy strategies to overcome these.

The second edition of *Adolescent Counseling* has 15 new chapters, along with case discussions regarding contemporary issues. These include media use, romantic relationships, coping with grief, anxiety, self-harm and eating disorders. Fundamentals of dialectical behavior therapy, motivational interviewing, trauma-informed care, cognitive behavior therapy, self-counseling, strengths, and life skills-based counseling have been included in this new edition. We have updated all the chapters of the first edition with recent advances in the field of counseling. Our dedicated team of experienced authors, comprising of pediatricians, psychologists, psychiatrists, and social workers through their lucid contributions have made adolescent counseling simple and doable in clinical practice. We hope that all gatekeepers of adolescent health counselors, teachers, social workers, healthcare professionals, parents, and policy makers—will enjoy reading this book and enable the adolescents under their care to achieve their potential and lead happy and fulfilling lives!

MKC Nair
Preeti M Galagali

Preface to the First Edition

Counseling is a popular term nowadays; but, unfortunately, it is probably not used for the right reasons. Counseling is not advising, but it is a learning process that enables personality development. Counseling is aimed at helping people make choices and act on them. In the present-day context, counseling may be required more for non-assertive adolescents and for those who have scholastic backwardness, specific behavioral problems and adjustment difficulties.

As part of the adjustment process at home and at school, adolescents constantly strive to satisfy their physiological or psychological motives; and when satisfaction is thwarted by internal and external barriers, frustration occurs. Conflicts, frustration and reaction towards unfavorable conditions arouse a general feeling of discomfort, causing disequilibrium in the adolescent mind and a whole set of defense mechanisms come into play, both positive and negative. In the counseling process, it is important to understand the above defense mechanisms, in order to fully appreciate the adolescent behavior and adjustment problems and use behavior modification as a remedial measure.

Compared to the state of affairs 25 years ago, we have achieved a lot in terms of material possessions, yet there is no happiness around among the young people. Happiness is an outstanding characteristic of mental health and it is an important prerequisite of good adjustment in life. The youngsters constantly seek expression of their potential; and those who are fortunate to have an enabling environment for developing and utilizing their capacities to the fullest are said to be progressing towards self-actualization.

Considering the enormous potential of the young people in the nation- building process, it is important that we nurture a whole new generation of motivated and self-actualizing youngsters. For this, adolescent mental health has to become a priority in the next five year plan. The National Health Mission (NHM) gives us the right opportunity to pilot community and school-based counseling programs. In the absence of clinical psychologis, as professional counselors in most part of the country, the pediatricians have to fill in the gap, with the help of trained counselors available locally. Hence, it may be worthwhile for all of us to try and understand the basic principles and practice of counseling. We do hope that this book, edited by adolescent pediatricians, child psychologists and social scientists' team, with over 35 years of child guidance and counseling experience, would serve the purpose.

MKC Nair
Indira MS
Babu George
Leena Sumaraj

Acknowledgments

I would like to thank Dr Babu George, Former Director; Dr Deepa Bhaskaran, Director-in-Charge; Dr Suresh Kumar G, Former Registrar; Ms Indira MS, Consultant Clinical Psychologist, Dr Mini K Paul, Consultant Clinical Psychologist; Suja S, Junior Programmer, and the other staff of Child Development Centre, Medical College Campus, Thiruvananthapuram, Kerala, India.

—MKC Nair

I would like to thank Dr Nalini (Clinical Psychologist); Dr Sharada Rangarajan (Special Educator), Bengaluru Adolescent Care and Counseling Centre, Karnataka, India, Dr Jagdish Chinappa, Cluster Head (Pediatrics), Manipal Hospital, Bengaluru; and Dr Gnanamurthy N, Director, Mother and Child Care Centre, Bengaluru, Karnataka, India.

—Preeti M Galagali

Contents

SECTION 1 Understanding Adolescent Behavior

SECTION 2 Fundamentals of Counseling

1 SECTION

Understanding Adolescent Behavior

1 CHAPTER

Introduction

MKC Nair, Harikumar SK

INTRODUCTION

Adolescence is a term that originated from "adolescere", a Latin word meaning to grow to maturity. Teenage is the period from 13 to 19 years of age and adolescence from 10 to 19 years of age (WHO). It is traditionally considered a stage of stress and storm, a dreaded age for others, as they are considered difficult to manage. Adolescence is described as a transitional age, the threshold of adulthood, a period of change and unrealism, and the time when the individual searches for identity. Adolescence is also the period when rapid changes occur in physical and sexual growth and cognitive development. The roles and responsibilities that are expected by society and the conflict between the actual expectation and achievement of the adolescents put them in a state of constant confusion and a sense of guilt and anxiety in some situations. Cognitive dissonance is a state of confusion and clouding that occurs in the thought process of a person. The stimulus that leads to the cognitive dissonance may vary from individual to individual depending on various social and environmental factors. In the population of different age groups, different issues are the priorities.

FACTORS THAT LEAD TO COGNITIVE DISSONANCE IN ADOLESCENTS

Physical Development

Adolescence is the period of rapid growth with development of breasts in girls, growth of facial hair in boys, and increase in body height and weight in both. It is more or less of the expected normal. The body image as such is a matter of concern to most. Yet, they may not be comfortable discussing these issues with relatives or teachers.

Emotional Development

In both girls and boys, because of the action of sex hormones, feminine and masculine behavioral patterns gradually set in; this may not be in tune with the expectations of parents, often forming the basis for conflict.

Sexual Development

Development of secondary sexual characters, menarche in girls and nocturnal emissions in boys, are sometimes factors that lead to conflict in cognition. The information on sex and sex-related matters that they gather from peers and other nonauthentic sources leads to a lot of misconceptions. Unnecessary fear and anxiety related to masturbation, a normal physiological sexual outlet, is an example in this regard.

Academic Achievement

Expectations on academic achievements from children of the adolescent age group, by parents and society, are very high. The competition is increasing, and the burden on adolescents for achievement in the academic field is also increasing. The admissions to various courses and opportunities for jobs have become highly competitive. The increasing number of suicides in connection with examination results is an indication of growing distress in the adolescent population with regard to academic expectations.

Interpersonal Relationships

Adolescence is the period during which a large number of friendships are made and broken. The expectation and understanding in these relationships are quite often very private and personal. Different people may have conflicting views on issues such as teenage love affairs, teenage sexuality, and more so about homosexual relationships, all affecting the development of normal interpersonal relationships.

Involvement in Social Issues

Enthusiasm and innovative ideas will always be the hallmark of the adolescent population. They will try to be involved in issues of social relevance. There may be situations when their ideas will not be in agreement with the popular social beliefs. This may result in conflicts with the establishment and elders. The situation where many adolescents are used by antisocial elements to get involved in destructive agitations, leading to campus fights and even murders, may be related to this situation. There have been increasing media reports on occasions of adolescents and youth being involved in serious criminal activities.

NEED FOR ADOLESCENT COUNSELING

Counseling may be required for nonassertive adolescents and for those who have adjustment difficulties, scholastic backwardness, character and personality disorders, and specific behavioral problems. By providing good-quality counseling by a competent and well-trained person, we will be able to establish an enhanced level of confidence and motivation in the adolescents. In this process, we are remodeling the perception, cognition, and expression of the younger generation aimed at a more productive and result-oriented working pattern. This process will be a joint working effort of the enthusiastic young generation and the technical and experienced professionals. In most of the situations, the availability of counseling services will ensure that the emotional disturbances of adolescents are properly attended to, before unhappiness and major adjustment problems crop up.

Characteristics of Adjustment and Happiness

- Life is an interplay between ourselves and the environment.
- There must be a need on the part of the individual to adjust.
- Adjustment is a continuous process.
- Adjustment is based on subjective feelings about ourselves rather than on how others see us.
- Adjustment requires that we respond selectively to different situations.

We all know that chronic unhappiness leads to maladjustment. The three essentials of happiness would be as follows:

1. *Acceptance:* Individuals who are accepted by others find it easy to like and accept themselves.

2. *Affection:* To receive affection, one must be able to show affection.
3. *Achievement:* Must be in an area that is valued by the social group with which he/she identifies.

During adolescence, the search for his/her identity is supreme and in the process of trying to achieve it, he/she comes into conflict with parental restrictions and societal norms. While the young adult is looking for intimacy in relations, the middle-aged is preoccupied with achievement. There should be no controversy regarding the fact that the ultimate goal of human life is self-actualization. The adolescent is capable of developing and ultimately reaching this stage, if he/she is helped to harmonize all aspects—cognition (knowledge), affect (feeling), and conation (action).

There are a number of areas in health and development in which adolescents have a lot of doubts and misconceptions. When it comes to issues related to sex and sexuality, the parent and teacher population also do not have clarity of thinking and comfort level to discuss these things. As adolescents get only unauthentic information on issues related to sexual aspects, many may end up being exploited sexually and physically. It is in this context that a good counselor should have clarity and authenticity of concepts, listening and empathizing skills, ability to approach the issue professionally, and the best skills in verbal and nonverbal communication.

BASIS OF COUNSELING

The fundamental philosophy of counseling is concern for the individual, faith in humanity, belief in the potentiality of human beings and groups, and institutions which embody values. There are differing views on human nature, on the one hand, saying it is essentially evil and, on the other hand, saying it is essentially good and that it is the environment that corrupts him/her. There is also a neutral viewpoint saying that good circumstances bring in good behavior and bad circumstances bring in bad behavior.

Counseling is the process of interpersonal interaction with the specific purpose of enabling a person to find his own solutions for his problems. The need for counseling arises when one really falls into the state of "cognitive dissonance".

It was Freud who first tried to explain the basic nature of people, as seeking pleasure and avoiding pain and the concept of the driving force or the basic energy of life called libido. According to him, "*id*" (primitive instinctual drives of aggression and sex) is the basis of human behavior. But then this "*id*" tends to come in conflict with "*superego*", the outgrowth of learning, the taboos and moral values of society. "*Ego*", develops to mediate between the demands of the "*id*" and the realities of the external world.

Concept of "Growth" and "Development"

For pediatricians, the term growth refers to quantitative changes: increase in size and structure. Not only does the child become bigger physically, but also the size and structure of the internal organs and the brain increase. The child grows mentally as well as physically. Development refers to qualitative and quantitative changes, all the physical and psychological changes, a human being undergoes in a lifetime from the moment of conception to death. It may be defined as a progressive series of orderly, coherent changes. "Progressive" signifies that the changes are directional and they lead forward rather than backward. "Orderly" and "coherent" suggest that there is a definite relationship between the changes taking place and those that preceded or will follow them. The human being is never static; from the moment of conception to the time of death, the person is undergoing changes. At every age, some of the changes that occur during the developmental process are just beginning, some are at their peak and some are in the process of decline, with both heredity and environmental factors playing an important role.

DEVELOPMENT OF SELF-IDENTITY

As the child enters the adolescent stage, he/she experiences a lot of stresses and strains as a result of the adjustment process to the rapid change in the physical and psychological systems. The crucial task of adolescence is the establishment of a sense of *ego* identity. If adolescents succeed in integrating roles in different situations, self-identity develops. If they are unable to establish a sense of stability in various aspects of their lives, it results in role confusion. During late adolescence and college years, this search for a sense of identity may lead to joining a variety of groups and a lot of confusion about career choice. If these issues are not resolved during this time, the individual may develop a sense of despair later in life.

The new responsibilities of early adulthood can create tension and frustration. An intimate relationship with someone else can provide relief. True intimacy is not possible without first achieving identity and gaining confidence in oneself. Some people develop a sense of intimacy, an acceptance of life's success and disappointments, and a sense of continuity throughout the life cycle. Other people remain isolated from family and friends, appear to survive on a fixed daily routine, and focus on both past disappointments and future death.

PSYCHOLOGICAL DEVELOPMENT

In the psychological parlor, the term growth refers to psychological development. All infants express their basic needs, and the degree to which these are satisfied is most important in establishing the child's trust in others. If the need is satisfied properly, the child develops confidence and basic trust is established, although not permanently. Any type of deprivation, anxiety, or rejection experienced at this stage will lead to a sense of mistrust. This is the basic psychological attitude acquired by the child. As children grow, they have a tendency to behave spontaneously and tend to acquire mastery over several things. They give their expressions through play. Children try to get recognition from others. If parents, teachers, or significant others restrict children's freedom or discourage them, it will have a negative effect on their personality. They will develop guilt or inferiority feelings that may affect their personal adjustment and interpersonal relationship in later life.

Motivation is a condition of needs or desire within the individual. It is the force that promotes an individual to act or behave. This force can be biological, as in the case of hunger or sleep needs, or it can be social, as in the need for achievement or the need for affiliation. Some motives appear to be innate; that is, they are programed. Others rely solely on learning and experiences within one's own external environment. Maslow's hierarchy of needs theory suggests that human needs appear to arrange themselves on a hierarchy, with physiological needs being the first to be satisfied and the desire to realize one's fullest potential the last. Starting with physiological needs (oxygen, water, food, and sex), it progresses to safety need, need for love and belonging, self-esteem need, and lastly self-actualization. Once the basic level of needs is met, human motivation is directed toward the next higher level needs.

According to Maslow, growth is a difficult and arduous process, and since there seems to be an innate tendency toward inertia and inactivity in the human species, a great deal of energy is needed to push forward. It is the child-rearing patterns that make the difference as to whether an individual will venture up the hierarchy. Although overprotectiveness and overindulgence hinder a child's ability to become strong and self-reliant, a loving, respectful environment with parents encouraging the development of skills and capabilities will give an individual the strength and confidence to climb the hierarchy. Maslow observed that those people who are self-actualizing are quite different psychologically than people who were not approaching their potential. Self-actualizing individuals are more spontaneous, accepting, problem-centered, autonomous, humorous, creative, and socially concerned than most others.

Personality, as defined by Allport, is "the dynamic organization within the individual of those psychophysical systems that determine his characteristic behavior and thought". Personality refers to the characteristic and unique ways in which an individual responds to the environment. Personality influences and determines all behavioral processes and provides a frame of reference for the psychological events occurring in the individual. Personality development takes place through various stages based on different aspects of development such as biological and psychosocial. During each stage, the child must resolve conflicts between needs or feelings and external obstacles. The satisfactory resolution of these conflicts leads to a healthy personality and a productive lifestyle.

COGNITIVE FACTORS

Cognitive process entails thinking, reasoning, problem-solving, and the use of language, imagining, fantasizing, and conceptualizing. This process mediates between environmental stimulation and the way in which people respond to that stimulation. Our thoughts, related images, expectations, attitudes/perceptions of past events influence our behavior; for example, a person who has an irrational belief that he/she must be loved, approved of, and accepted by everyone is more likely to face rejection and depression as compared to another who does not have this belief. Hence, it becomes important to assess the client's "internal dialogue" and the way in which this relates to his/her presenting problem.

According to cognitive developmental theory, behavior reflects the emergence of various cognitive structures, organized units, or patterns of thinking that influence how the child interprets experience. Thinking pertains to the organization and manipulation of ideas, images, and concepts that come through learning and experience. How one thinks depends on biological development and the environmental forces that are confronted. Generally, there are two kinds of thinking namely, directed and nondirected.

1. Directed thinking pertains to reasoning and problem-solving procedures aimed at meeting specific goals.
2. Nondirected thinking refers to daydreaming, free association, fantasy, and other flowing uncontrolled activity.

Schemes for Thinking

Jean Piaget's vision of human development was based on two overriding assumptions about intelligence. It is a form of biological adaptation and becomes organized as the individual interacts with the external world. Thus, thinking exhibits two inborn qualities. The first is adaptation, a tendency to adjust oneself to or become more attuned to the conditions imposed by the environment. The second is organization, a tendency for intellectual structures and processes to become more systematic and coherent. The basic mental structure in Piaget's theory is a scheme, a coordinated and systematic pattern of action or way of reasoning. A scheme is a kind of template for acting or thinking applied to similar classes of objects or situations.

- The infant's schemes are limited to patterns of action applied to objects e.g., sucking, grasping, shaking, and so forth.
- The older child's schemes will often involve mental processes and be far more complex as he or she reasons about such

things as classes of objects, number or spatial relations, and by adolescence, the meaning of life and the origin of the universe.

- At all levels of development, individuals apply schemes as a means of interacting with the environment. Individuals assimilate ideas or fit them into existing schemes of knowledge, and they also make accommodations, that is, change their perceptions and verbal stimulation from the environment.

Piaget believed that schemes change through two complementary processes.

Assimilation refers to the process of interpreting an experience in terms of current ways of understanding things.

Accommodation refers to the modifications in behavior and thinking that take place, when the old ways of understanding the schemes no longer fit. For Piaget, assimilation and accommodation are complementary aspects of all psychological activities, processes engaged in a constant tug of war in the never-ending goal of acquiring understanding.

Equilibration is the process by which assimilation and accommodation bring about more organized and powerful schemes for thinking.

DEFINITION OF COUNSELING

Pepinsky and Pepinsky state that "counseling is a process involving an interaction between a counselor and a client in a private setting, with the purpose of helping the client change his/her behavior, so that a satisfactory resolution of needs may be obtained". Arbuckle distinguishes guidance from counseling by equating guidance with the distributive phase where the focus is on one's educational, vocational, or occupational problems, while counseling is associated with the adjustment phase in which the emphasis is on social, personal, or emotional problems of the individual. Counseling may be for three purposes, namely:

1. Remedial role, e.g., marital counseling
2. Preventive role, e.g., suicide prevention program
3. Educative and developmental role, e.g., family life education programs

GOALS OF COUNSELING

- Resolution of problems
- Improving personal effectiveness—enhancing coping skills
- Decision making—avoiding impulsive actions, reducing the possibility of error
- Modification of behavior—facilitating behavior change and removal of undesirable behavior
- Differentiating "normal" and "abnormal" behavior
- Improving relationships
- Facilitating client potential
- Improving scholastic achievement in adolescents
- Promoting mental health—through school teen clubs

Points to Be Emphasized in Counseling

- Maintaining the client's adaptive patterns
- Modifying maladaptive patterns
- Enhancing the motivation of the client
- Identifying the etiology of the problem
- Promoting growth—personal progress
- Promoting problem solving—becoming more assertive
- Avoiding frustration and bringing in happiness

QUALITIES OF A COUNSELOR

A successful counselor would be interested in helping people and thus deriving a lot of satisfaction from it. He/she would have perceptual sensitivity, meaning the capacity to pick up cues and clues. It is not necessary that the counselor should be "perfectly adjusted" to be a good counselor, but all the same must be a genuine person, with a lot of personal security and a high comfort level. The counselor has to keep in mind the concept of individual freedom, liberty, and sovereignty of the counselee and learn to respect the client's values, religious beliefs, customs, etc. A good counselor must have the following qualities:

- Listening more than talking
- Empathy not sympathy
- Professionalism—knowledge, skill, attitude

- Effective communication
- Constructive in approach
- Congruent in nature
- Confidentiality at all times
- Accepting one's freedom of choice

TYPES OF COUNSELING

- Directive counseling—counselor plays a leading role
- Nondirective counseling—the counselee plays a predominant role
- Eclectic counseling—combination of directive, nondirective, and other approaches
- Group counseling—groups help him/her to understand and solve problems in the context of the social reality

APPROACHES TO COUNSELING

Counseling is a personal meeting of two individuals: the counselee, who has a problem and needs assistance, and the counselor who assists in analyzing and understanding the problem, thus equipping the counselee for self-help. The problems of the counselee may be emotional, psychological, social, or academic.

Psychoanalytic Approach to Counseling

Freudian theory of personality is built on the premise that the mind is topographical and dynamic. In the conscious mind, thoughts, ideas, and images are present that are accessible but lie above the threshold of awareness. Directly below this level is the preconscious mind, which houses information just beneath the surface of awareness, which is easily brought to consciousness if needed. Another important realm of mind is the unconscious, the part that is outside awareness, the knowledge of which is inferred through dreams, slips of the tongue, fantasies, and symptoms of mental disorder.

Sigmund Freud's theory of psychoanalysis regards human personality as significantly influenced by two basic forces, sex and aggression, constantly seeking expression in the individual. These impulses, according to the theory, are part of our inborn nature and the denial of their expression as often required by society does not result in their disappearance. Instead, they find release in a disguised form. This process of denial and disguised expression is called unconscious motives. It is the central idea in psychoanalytic theory, and it is most relevant to childhood, when the personality is being formed. Conflicts and frustration at this age, especially concerning sex and aggression, can have a significant and unexpected influence later on the adult personality. As mentioned earlier, the building blocks of personality in psychoanalytic theory consist of three systems or forces: *id, ego,* and *superego*. The *id* is the storehouse of impulses and unconscious drives and operates on the pleasure principle. The *ego* works on the reality principle that often requires a suspension of the pleasure principle, depending on the circumstances in the environment. The *superego* corresponds to what we call commonly as the conscience, which of course will depend on the standards of the society or forces outside the individual.

Behavioral Approach to Counseling

Learning theory and the behavioral point of view emphasize that there are three broad assumptions about the nature of a person.

Behavior is learned by the building up of associations: Complexity can be understood in terms of the building up and joining together of simple associative bonds between something that occurs in the environment and the individual's response to it.

People basically seek to obtain pleasure and avoid pain: A behavior, which in a given situation produces satisfaction, becomes associated with that situation and is likely to recur when the situation recurs. Conversely, any behavior/act that produces discomfort becomes dissociated with the situation.

Behavior is basically environmentally determined: Environment plays an important role in determining behavior.

In the behavioral approach, psychological problems are regarded as learned responses that have harmful consequences for the individual or for his or her environment. Generally, behavior therapy techniques are based on the principles of learning and conditioning—classical and operant conditioning. The classical conditioning procedure suggests that much abnormal behavior is the result of conditioning responses to inappropriate stimuli. When an undesirable response is elicited too frequently or by too wide a range of stimuli, therapy based on classical conditioning is directed at helping the client unlearn the connection and replace the old conditioned response with a more adaptive response. Therapies based on operant conditioning are used in order to establish and maintain an appropriate contingency relationship so that the desired behavior is rewarded. A reinforcer increases the probability of the responses it follows. Behavior is brought under the control of the therapist through the manipulation of schedules of reinforcement.

Humanistic Approach to Counseling

Carl Rogers's humanistic approach to counseling is based on the concept that many individuals are not in touch with their true selves. They have a false self-image and the behaviors they exhibit confirm this inaccuracy. The humanistic approach states that human beings among all species have a special capacity for self-direction, meaning the capacity for guiding their own lives and the potential for change. There is an emphasis on human uniqueness and special endowments, which promote self-direction. According to the humanists, individuals are driven by a need for self-actualization tendency, an inborn predisposition to develop and use all the capacities that maintain, enhance, and fulfill the organism. It includes not only primary drives but also drives toward competency and mastery. In the humanistic approach, there is no inherently negative motive. Actualization is exclusively a positive motive. Antisocial behavior occurs only when the actualizing tendency is adversely influenced by environmental circumstances. As children grow, parents and others react to their behavior, sometimes with disapproval and sometimes in a positive way. They thus learn to regard some of their actions or feelings as unworthy and react by destroying or denying them.

Maslow and the Motivation Hierarchy

The five needs in Maslow's motivational hierarchy are (1) physiological, (2) safety-security, (3) belongingness, (4) self-esteem, and (5) self-actualization. Operational definitions were developed from Maslow's theory of motivation. Strong support for the validity and reliability of all five needs measures was obtained from psychometric tests of the scales conducted on questionnaire results from 386 adult respondents from the general population. Although family support, traditional values, and life satisfaction had significant positive correlations with the satisfaction of all five needs, the anxiety/worry facet of neuroticism had significant negative correlations with the satisfaction of all the needs.

Neurodevelopment in adolescence: In adolescence, the brain undergoes rapid changes. According to the "use it or lose it" principle, the neuronal connections that are used the most get stronger, whereas those that are not used get pruned off or disappear. Hence, adolescents who are motivated and counseled to adopt a healthy lifestyle (e.g., adequate nutrition, physical activity, sleep, stress management techniques, healthy media use) continue to follow it over the entire life span and do not suffer from noncommunicable diseases. As puberty begins, the emotional center (limbic system) and reward center of the brain mature, while the executive center (prefrontal cortex) is fully developed (myelinated) only in the late twenties. This results in heightened emotions, impulsivity, mood swings, and sensation-seeking behavior in adolescence. Adolescents need to learn life skills for socioemotional regulation. Parents, teachers, and counselors should facilitate this learning through role modeling, empathetic interaction, and counseling. Individuals from 10 to 24 years are grouped together as adolescents and young adults (AYA) or young people as they are vulnerable to similar health risks due to a developing brain. Neurodevelopment is influenced by genetics, temperament, chronic medical disorders, parental and school connectivity, spirituality, media use, governmental health policies, pollution, and geopolitical climate. The brain development is impaired in adolescents who have adverse childhood experiences and live in poverty. They may present with problem behaviors and physical and mental disorders during adolescence.

CONCLUSION

Adolescence is a transitional phase of life between childhood and adulthood characterised by rapid changes in the biopsychosocial domains. These changes can result in cognitive dissonance in adolescence. Counseling helps to resolves this dissonance and eases mental distress. There are many schools and approaches to counselling like psychoanalytic, behavioral, humanistic, eclectic etc. Counselors should adopt a genuine patient centric empathetic attitude to build a therapeutic alliance with the adolescent. Counseling in adolescence can promote a healthy lifestyle and well being over the entire lifespan.

SUGGESTED READING

1. Bukatko D, Daehler MW. Child Development – A Thematic Approach, 3rd edition. New York: Houghton Mifflin Harcourt Company; 1998.
2. Fernald LD, Fernald PS. Introduction to Psychology, 5th edition. New Delhi: AITBS Publishers and Distributors; 1999.
3. Hurlock EB. Child Development. New York: McGraw-Hill; 1978.
4. Pervin LA. Personality: Theory and Research, 4th edition. New York: John Wiley and Sons, Inc.; 1984.
5. Sharma E, Ravi GS, Kumar K, Thennarasu K, Heron J, Hickman M, et al. Growth trajectories for executive and social cognitive abilities in an Indian population sample: impact of demographic and psychosocial determinants. Asian J Psychiatr. 2023;82:103475.
6. Taormina RJ, Gao JH. Maslow and the motivation hierarchy: measuring satisfaction of the needs. Am J Psychol. 2013;126(2):155-77.

2 CHAPTER

Developmental Theories

Sonny Jose

INTRODUCTION

One may perhaps wonder the relevance of theories to practice. The Greek word *theoros* translates as "spectator". Theory is a way of looking at or surveying a field of evidence with a view of extracting principles from it. First and foremost, theories give us a better understanding of the problems presented by the clients. In fact, such an understanding helps the counselor/therapist evolve an effective treatment strategy. Theoretical bases also provide a common platform for members of a medical team in understanding the client's problem as well as designing a treatment based on the approach taken in comprehending the client's problem. Finally, they help team members in defining their individual roles and share the same as part of a medical team.

Each individual is unique in terms of his/her biopsychosocial experience. As a professional counselor or a social worker, the therapist is confronted by cases with a lot of diversities—gender, age, culture, experience, etc. In order to understand and deal with these, the therapist must have a sound grounding regarding the various developmental stages that an individual undergoes during his or her life span. In this chapter, the author intends to specifically discuss various theories pertaining to development during a life span. When discussing any type of development, most theorists break it down into specific stages. These stages are typically progressive. In other words, you must pass through one stage, before you can get to the next. Think about how you learned to run: first, you had to learn to crawl, then you learnt to walk, and finally you developed the skills needed for running. Without the first two stages, running would be impossible.

Let us now discuss the most prominent stage theories with regard to cognitive development, social development, and moral development.

The following text offers an overview of development according to the principles of psychology.

PIAGET'S STAGES OF COGNITIVE DEVELOPMENT

Probably the most cited theory regarding cognitive development in children is the theory by Jean Piaget. As with all stage theories, Piaget's theory of cognitive development maintains that children go through specific stages as their intellect and ability to see relationships mature. These stages are completed universally in a fixed order by all children. The age range, however, may vary from child to child.

Sensorimotor Stage (0–2 Years)

This stage occurs between the ages of birth and 2 years, as infants begin to understand the information entering their sense and develop the ability to interact with the world. During this stage, the children learn to manipulate objects, although they fail to understand the permanency of these objects, if not within their current sensory perception. In other words, once an object is removed from the child's view, he or she is unable to understand that the object still exists.

Object Permanency

The major achievement during this stage is the acquisition of object permanency, the ability to understand that these objects do in fact continue to exist in spite of not being visible. This includes the child's ability to understand that when the mother leaves the room, she will eventually return, resulting in an increased sense of safety and security. Object permanency occurs toward the end of this stage and represents the child's ability to maintain a mental image of the object (or person) in its absence.

Preoperational Stage (2–7 Years)

- *Transductive thought:* Piaget describes children in this age range as using transductive thought, a form of prelogical thought, which connects two observable events that have occurred contiguously and the child has associated them, as if there were a logical connection between them. During this stage, the development of language occurs at a rapid pace. Children learn how to interact with their environment in a more complex manner through the use of words and images.

- *Egocentrism:* The child believes that everyone else sees the world the same way that he/she does. Thus, a child during this stage fails to understand the differences in perception and believes that inanimate objects have the same perceptions he/she does, such as seeing things, feeling, hearing, and his/her sense of touch.
- *Conservation:* It is the ability to understand that quantity does not change even if the shape changes. In other words, if a short and wide glass beaker of water is poured into a tall and thin glass beaker, children in this stage will perceive the taller glass beaker as having more water. They attribute this to the height. This is due to the child's inability to understand reversibility and to focus on only one aspect of a stimulus (termed centration), such as height, as opposed to understanding other aspects, such as glass width or even volume.

Concrete Operations Stage (7–12 Years)

Occurring between ages 7 and about 12 years, the third stage of cognitive development is marked by a gradual decrease in centristic thought and the increased ability to include more than one aspect of a stimulus.

- *Inductive thought:* Now, children can understand the concept of grouping, i.e., they are capable of comprehending that both a small dog and a large dog are still dogs or those coins and rupee notes are part of the bigger concept of money.
- *Reversibility and conservation:* Due to the acquisition of these, they begin to comprehend volume (vs. weight or mass) and depth (vs. length). Thus, they start to manipulate Lego blocks to create structures, dismantle them, and reassemble these to create still newer ones. Having comprehended the concept of mass, they would be able to discriminate that a mass of dough in a ball form can be rolled into a chapati and vice versa.

Unfortunately, they can apply this new understanding only to concrete objects (those they have actually experienced). In other words, since abstract thinking has not yet developed, imagined objects or those they have not seen, heard, or touched continue to remain somewhat mystical to these children.

Formal Operations Stage (12 Years and Above)

During the final stage of cognitive development (from age 12 years and beyond), the individual begins to develop a more abstract view of the world.

Deductive Thought

The child in the formal operational stage is able to think both inductively and deductively, although he/she may resort to more primitive modes of thought from time to time. Children are able to apply reversibility and conservation to both real and imagined situations as well as abstract social situations. They also develop an increased understanding of the functional world and the idea of cause and effect. By teenage, they are able to develop their own theories about the world. Most children achieve this stage, although failure to do so has been associated with lower intelligence.

ERIKSON'S STAGES OF PSYCHOSOCIAL DEVELOPMENT

Like Piaget, Erik Erikson maintained that children develop in a predetermined sequence. Instead of focusing on cognitive development, however, he took interest in how children socialize and how this affected their sense of self. Erikson's theory of psychosocial development perceived psychosocial development as happening in eight distinct stages, each with two possible outcomes. According to this theory, successful completion of each stage results in a healthy personality and successful interactions with others, while failure results in a reduced ability to complete further stages and therefore an unhealthy personality and poor sense of self. Nevertheless, these stages can be resolved successfully at a later time.

Stage 1: Trust Versus Mistrust (0–1 Year)

From the time of birth up to 1 year, children begin to learn the ability to trust others based on the consistency and warmth of care received from their caregiver(s). If the trust develops successfully, the children feel confident and secure, and they feel safe even when threatened. Unsuccessful completion of this stage can result in an inability to trust others, and therefore they suffer from a sense of insecurity and fear about the inconsistencies in the world. It may result in anxiety, heightened insecurity, and an overwhelming feeling of mistrust in the world around them.

Stage 2: Autonomy Versus Shame and Doubt (1–3 Years)

Between the ages of 1 and 3 years, children begin to assert their independence, by walking away from the mother, choosing and picking up toys to play with, and making choices about what they like to wear or eat, etc. Similarly, they attempt to walk, spoon the food, brush the teeth, gain bladder and bowel control, etc., by trial and error. If children in this stage are encouraged and supported in their attempts to gain independence, they become more confident and secure in their own ability to survive in the world. If children are criticized, overly controlled, or not given the opportunity to assert themselves, they begin to feel inadequate in their ability to survive. Consequently, they may become overly dependent upon others, lack self-esteem, and feel a sense of shame or doubt in their own abilities.

Stage 3: Initiative Versus Guilt (3–6 Years)

Around age 3 years and continuing to age 6 years, children assert themselves more frequently. During this age, the child moves out from the protected home environment into the preschool environment. Being at school presents them with opportunities to plan activities, make up games, and initiate activities with others mostly of the same age group. Given such opportunities, children develop a sense of initiative and feel secure in their ability to handle others, lead as well as make decisions. Conversely, if this initiative is stalled through either criticism or control, children develop a sense of guilt. Consequently, they may feel that they are "unwanted" and are a nuisance to others. Such children therefore remain followers, lacking in self-initiative or leadership.

Stage 4: Industry Versus Inferiority (6–12 Years)

During "school age", i.e., from age 6 years to puberty, children begin to develop a sense of pride in their accomplishments. They initiate projects, see them through to completion, and feel good about what they have achieved. During this time, teachers play an increased role in the child's development especially acquiring the 3Rs—reading, writing, and arithmetic. If children are encouraged and reinforced for their initiative, they begin to feel industrious and confident in their ability to achieve goals. On the other hand, if such initiatives are not encouraged, or if it they are restricted by parents or teachers, then the child begins to feel inferior, seriously doubting his/her own abilities and therefore may fail to achieve his/her potential.

Stage 5: Identity Versus Role Confusion (13–19 Years)

Teenage is the period of transition from childhood to adulthood. During this stage, children generally become more independent. During this phase, individuals generally get into conflicts with their parents and authority figures over decisions. This need only be considered as a transient phase, during which an attempt is made to gain emancipation psychologically from the parent figures. More importantly, they begin to look at the future in terms of a career, relationships, family, sexual orientation, etc. During this period, they explore all possibilities and begin to construct their own identity based on the outcome of these explorations. This sense of "who they are" can be hindered, resulting in a sense of confusion (I don't know what I want to be when I grow up) about themselves and their role in the world.

Stage 6: Intimacy Versus Isolation (Young Adulthood)

Occurring in young adulthood, we begin to share ourselves more intimately with others. We explore relationships leading toward longer-term commitments with someone other than family members. Such commitments may be in the form of marriage, work, or organizations. Successful achievement of these can lead to comfortable relationships and a sense of commitment, safety, and care within a relationship. Avoiding intimacy and fearing commitment and relationships can lead to isolation, loneliness, and sometimes depression.

Stage 7: Generativity Versus Stagnation (Middle Adulthood)

During middle adulthood, we establish our careers, settle down within a relationship, begin our own families, and, thus, develop a sense of being part of the bigger picture. We give back to society through raising our children, being productive at work, and becoming involved in community activities and civic organizations. By failing to achieve these objectives, we become stagnant and feel unproductive.

Stage 8: Ego Integrity Versus Despair (Senior Citizens)

As we grow older and become senior citizens, we tend to slow down in terms of productivity and finally disengage from life activities. Left with little resources and nothing much to do, the individual attempts to explore life as a retired person. It is during this time that we contemplate our accomplishments. If we see ourselves as leading a successful life, we develop integrity. If we see our lives as unproductive, feel guilt about our past, or feel that we did not accomplish our life goals, we become dissatisfied with life and develop despair, often leading to depression and hopelessness.

FREUD'S STAGES OF PSYCHOSEXUAL DEVELOPMENT

Sigmund Freud is probably the most well-known theorist when it comes to the development of personality. Freud's stages of psychosexual development are, like other stage theories, completed in a predetermined sequence and can result in either successful achievement of a healthy personality or failure, leading to an unhealthy personality. This theory is probably the most well-known as well as the most controversial, as Freud believed that we develop through stages based upon a particular erogenous zone. Any sort of failure during each stage leads the child to become fixated on that particular erogenous zone, precipitating an over- or underindulgence once he/she becomes an adult.

Stage 1: Oral Stage (0–18 Months)

During the oral stage, the child is focused on oral pleasures (sucking). Too much or too little gratification can result in an "oral fixation" or "oral personality", which is evidenced by a preoccupation with oral activities. Freud postulated that such type of personality may have a stronger tendency to smoke, drink alcohol, overeat, or bite his/her nails. Personality-wise, these individuals may become overly dependent upon others, gullible, and perpetual followers. On the other hand, they may also fight these urges and develop pessimism and become hypercritical and aggressive toward others.

Stage 2: Anal Stage (18–36 Months)

The child's focus of pleasure in this stage is on eliminating and retaining feces. Through society's pressure, mainly via parents, the child has to learn to control anal stimulation. In terms of personality, the after-effects of an anal fixation during this stage can result in an obsession with cleanliness, perfection, and control (anal retentive). On the opposite end of the spectrum, he/she may become messy and disorganized (anal expulsive).

Stage 3: Phallic Stage (3–6 Years)

During this stage, the erogenous zone switches to the genitals. Freud believed that during this stage, a boy develops unconscious sexual desires for his mother. Because of this, he finds a rival in his father and sees him as competition for the mother's affection. However, fully aware of the father's domination, boys also develop a fear that their father will punish them for these feelings, by castrating them (castration anxiety). This group of feelings is known as "Oedipus complex", named after the Greek mythological figure, who accidentally killed his father and married his mother.

As if to balance off, later it was added that girls go through a similar situation. It was described that girls develop an unconscious sexual attraction for their father as a way of placating the love the father was seen to give to the mother. Although Freud strongly disagreed with this, it has been termed the "Electra complex" by more recent psychoanalysts.

According to Freud, out of fear of castration and due to the strong competition of his father, the boy eventually decides to identify with him rather than fight him. By identifying with his father, the boy develops masculine characteristics and identifies himself as a male and represses his sexual feelings toward his mother. A fixation at this stage could result in sexual deviancies (both overindulging and avoidance) and weak or confused sexual identity according to psychoanalysts.

Stage 4: Latency Stage (6–12 Years)

During this stage, sexual urges remain repressed. Children during this stage spend most of their time interacting and playing mostly with same-sex peers.

Stage 5: Genital Stage (Puberty On)

The final stage of psychosexual development begins at the start of puberty when sexual urges are once again awakened. Through the lessons learned during the previous stages, adolescents direct their sexual urges onto opposite-sex peers, with the primary focus of pleasure being on the genitals.

FREUD'S STRUCTURAL AND TOPOGRAPHICAL MODELS OF PERSONALITY

Sigmund Freud's theory and his writings on psychosexual development set the groundwork for how our personalities developed. He also believed that different driving forces develop during each of these stages which play an important role in how we interact with the world.

Structural Model (Id, Ego, and Superego)

According to Freud, we are born with our id. The id is an important part of our personality because as newborns, it allows us to meet our basic needs. Freud believed that the id operated based on the pleasure principle (immediate satiation). In other words, the id wants and does whatever it feels good at any time, with no consideration for the reality of the situation. When a child is hungry, the id wants food, and therefore the child cries. When the child needs to be changed, the id makes him/her cry. When the child is uncomfortable, in pain, too hot, too cold, or just wants attention, the id speaks up until his/her needs are met. The id does not care about reality or about the needs of anyone else, but only about its own satisfaction. If you think about it, babies are not real considerate of their parents' wishes. They have no care for time, whether their parents are sleeping, relaxing, eating dinner, or bathing. When the id wants something, nothing else is important.

Within the next 3 years, as the child interacts more and more with the world, the second part of the personality begins to differentiate and develop. Freud called this part the ego. The ego operates based on the reality principle. It understands that other people have needs and desires and that sometimes being impulsive or selfish can hurt us in the long run. It is the ego's job to meet the needs of the id, while taking into consideration the reality of the situation.

By the age of 5 years, or the end of the phallic stage of development, the superego develops. The superego is the moral part of us and develops from the moral and ethical restraints placed on us by our caregivers. Many equate the superego with the conscience, as it dictates our belief of right and wrong.

In a healthy person, according to Freud, the ego is the strongest so that it can satisfy the needs of the id, not upset the superego, and still take into consideration the reality of every situation. Not an easy job by any means, but if the id gets too strong, impulses and self-gratification take over the person's life. If the superego becomes very strong, the person would be driven by rigid morals and would be judgmental and unbending in his/her interactions with the world. We shall learn how the ego maintains control as we continue to proceed.

TOPOGRAPHICAL MODEL

Topographically, Freud structures the mind into three distinct domains—the conscious, the unconscious, and the preconscious. Freud believed that the majority of what we experience in our lives, the underlying emotions, beliefs, feelings, and impulses are not available to us at a conscious level. He believed that most of what drives us is buried in our unconscious. Most socially unacceptable and undesirable instincts are both pushed down into the unconscious, out of our awareness, due to the extreme anxiety they cause. However, even when buried there, they continue to impact us by occasionally popping into the conscious realm, at times quite dramatically.

The role of the unconscious is only one part of the model. Freud also believed that everything we are aware of is stored in our conscious. Our conscious makes up a very small part of who we are. In other words, at any given time, we are aware of only a very small part of what makes up our personality; most of what we are is buried and remains inaccessible.

The final part is the preconscious or subconscious. This is the part of us that we can access if prompted but is not in our active conscious. It is right below the surface but still buried somewhat unless we search for it. Information such as our telephone number, some childhood memories, or the name of our best childhood friend is stored in the preconscious.

Because the unconscious is so large, and because we are aware of only the very small conscious at any given time, this theory has been likened to an iceberg, where the vast majority is buried beneath the water surface. The water, by the way, would represent everything that we are not aware of and have not experienced and, and that has not been integrated into our personalities **(Fig. 1)**.

EGO DEFENSE MECHANISMS

We stated earlier that the ego's job was to satisfy the id's impulses, not offend the moralistic character of the superego, while still taking into consideration the reality of the situation. We also stated that this was not an easy job. Think of the id as the wild horse and the superego as the rider. We do not want either one to get too strong. So, a rein is used in order to regulate or control both of them. The ego, likened to the rein, takes an appropriate decision after having listened to their perspectives. This decision is the ego talking and looking for that healthy balance.

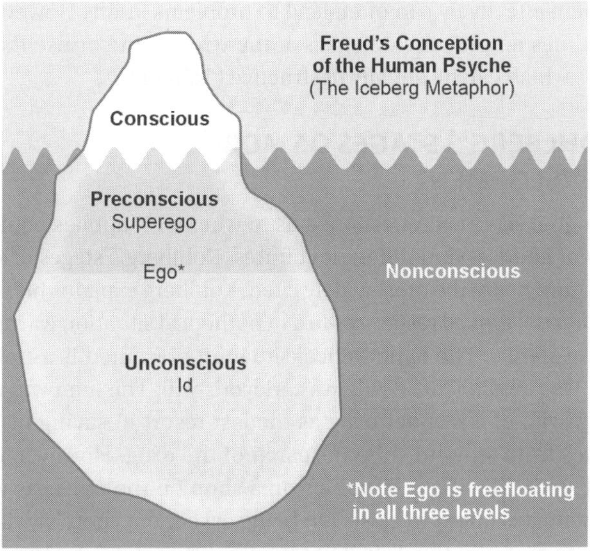

Fig. 1: Freud's topographic depiction of the human mind—preconscious, conscious, and unconscious—in relation with the ego states—id, ego, and superego.

Before we can talk more about this, we need to understand what drives the id, ego, and superego. According to Freud, we only have two drives: Sex and aggression. In other words, everything we do is motivated by one of these two drives. Sex, also called Eros or the life force, represents our drive (instinct) to live, prosper, and produce offspring. Aggression, also called Thanatos or our death force, represents our need to stay alive and stave off threats to our existence, our power, and our prosperity.

There are times when the ego has a difficult time satisfying both the id and the superego. Then the ego utilizes certain tools to help defend the ego and get its job done as the mediator. These are called ego defense mechanisms or defenses. When the ego has a difficult time making both the id and the superego happy, it will employ one or more of these defenses listed in the following text.

Ego defenses are not necessarily unhealthy as you can see by the above example. In fact, the lack of these defenses or the inability to use them effectively can often lead to problems in life. However, we sometimes employ the defenses at the wrong time or use them in excess, which can be equally destructive **(Table 1)**.

KOHLBERG'S STAGES OF MORAL DEVELOPMENT

Although it has been questioned as to whether it applies equally to different genders and different cultures, Kohlberg's stages of moral development are the most widely cited. Kohlberg explains his theory based on the typical responses to a hypothetical situation warranting a moral stance. The hypothetical situation presented is as follows: There was a man whose wife was grievously ill. The man was asked to get a vial of a wonder drug as the last resort in saving his wife. He goes from shop to shop in search of the drug. However, it was out of stock. He finally stumbles on a shop on the outskirts where the chemist is about to close. On being asked, the chemist willingly agrees to give him the drug, but for an exorbitant price. Despite the man pleading and explaining his predicament, the chemist refuses to part with the drug. He sticks to his price and closes down the shop.

The subjects were asked whether the man should steal the drug. Kohlberg later analyzed the responses of the subjects based on their age grouping. He classified the development of morality into three levels, each of which was further divided into two substages.

Preconventional Level (up to Age 9 Years): Self-Focused Morality

Here, the moral decisions are based on their limited experiences within their own world—themselves and their family.

Punishment-and-Obedience Orientation

Morality is defined as obeying rules and avoiding negative consequences. Children in this stage see rules set, typically by parents, as defining moral law. The typical response of a child during this stage would be, "The man should steal the drug because if he lets his wife die, he would be in great trouble". or "He will be blamed for not spending money on her".

TABLE 1: Various ego defense mechanisms with illustrations.

Description	***Example***
Denial: Arguing against an anxiety-provoking stimulus by stating it does not exist	Denying that the physician's diagnosis of cancer is correct and seeking a second opinion
Displacement: Taking out impulses on a less threatening target	Slamming a door instead of hitting a person, yelling at spouse after an argument with the boss
Intellectualization: Avoiding unacceptable emotions by focusing on the intellectual aspects	Focusing on the details of a funeral as opposed to the sadness and grief
Projection: Attributing unacceptable impulses in oneself to someone else	When losing an argument, one states "You're just stupid" or blame someone for a failure
Rationalization: Supplying a logical or rational reason as opposed to the real reason	When fired because of poor performance, alleging that it was because one did not kiss the boss
Reaction formation: Taking the opposite belief because the true belief causes anxiety	Having a bias against a particular race or culture and then embracing that race or culture to the other extreme
Regression: Returning to a previous stage of development	• Sitting in a corner and crying after hearing bad news • Throwing a temper tantrum when one do not get his/her way
Repression: Pulling into the unconscious	Being amnesic by eliminating from one's own consciousness the trauma of sexual abuse during childhood
Sublimation: Acting out unacceptable impulses in a socially acceptable way	• Sublimating aggressive impulses toward a career as a boxer • Becoming a surgeon because of one's desire to cut • Lifting weights to release "pent-up" energy
Suppression: Pushing into the unconscious	Trying to forget something that causes anxiety

Source: Adapted from Zastrow C. Practice of Social Work. New York: Brookes and Cole; 1994.

Naïve Hedonistic Orientation

During this stage, the child would do what he/she thinks is right, based on his/her own liking. Here, that which satisfies the child's own needs is seen as good and moral; the response would correspondingly be something like, e.g., "The man shouldn't steal the drug unless he is so crazy about his wife. He is running a terrible risk stealing the drug".

Conventional Level (Age 9 Years to Adolescence): Other Focused Morality

Gradually, as the child grows up and attends school, he/she becomes exposed to a larger circle of people. This transition forces him/her to consider the viewpoints of others in determining right and wrong.

Good-Boy/-Girl Orientation

Children begin to understand what is expected of them by their parents, teachers, etc. Morality is seen as satisfying the expectations of these significant persons; for example, "It is OK to steal the drug because no one will ever think you are bad if you did so. If you don't and let your wife die, you will never be able to look anyone in their face".

Social Order–Maintaining Orientation

During adolescence, the individual tends to become more idealistic. Here, fulfilling obligations as well as following expectations is seen as moral law for children in this stage. For example, "The man should steal the drug since he took a vow to stand by his wife in marriage. It is wrong to steal, so he should be expected to pay for his actions". or "It is natural for a man to save his wife's life, yet it is also wrong to steal. Even if his wife is dying that is not enough excuse to steal. If everyone did this the society would cease to exist".

Postconventional Level (Adulthood)

Higher Focused Morality

As the individual graduates into adulthood, he/she becomes capable of abstraction. Subsequently, he/she tends to be more realistic, objective, and universal in his/her thinking.

Social Contract/Legalistic Orientation

As adults, we begin to understand that people have different opinions about morality and that rules and laws vary from group to group and culture to culture. Morality is seen as upholding the values of one's group or culture. For example, "Although stealing is against the law, stealing the drug is justified. By doing so he saves his wife's life; life is more important than property" or "There is a law against stealing which represents the will of the majority. By living in a society he agrees to abide by the law, so stealing is a violation of this agreement".

Universal Ethical Principle Orientation

Understanding their own personal beliefs allows adults to judge themselves and others based on higher levels of morality. During this stage, judging on what is right and wrong is based more on the circumstances surrounding an action. Basics of morality are the foundation with independent thought playing an important role, e.g., the man may justify his stealing drugs to save his wife's life as it falls within his belief system of valuing and respecting a human life. On the other hand, even if the man is not blamed by others, he may believe that he has done wrong as he has has violated his own standards of honesty. So the man's independent thoughts will govern the judgment of his actions.

THE *ASHRAMAS*

Manu Dharma-Sastra proposes a very simple and logical way of looking at the developments occurring during a life span. It talks of the *Chatur* (four) *ashramas—Brahmacharya ashrama, Grihastha ashrama, Vanaprastha ashrama*, and *Sannyasa ashram. Brahmacharya ashrama* is the stage describing the phase from birth to adolescence. Considered the best stage of molding one's character, the child attaches herself/himself to a teacher in a *Gurukula*. During this stage, the experienced teacher (the *guru*) imparts knowledge and teaches the child the basic skills necessary for a successful life. Following the onset of puberty and adolescence, the child acquires the reproductive capacity and there is a sexual awakening.

The *Brahmachari* is now ready for marital life, known as *Grihastha ashrama*. During this stage, the individual embraces materialism. In this phase, the individual enjoys the bliss of marital life, procreates to have progeny (as a prerequisite for *Moksha*), and acquires *dravya* necessary to sustain the immediate generation. *Vanaprastha*, quite similar to middle age, is the stage during which the couple partially withdraws from the ways of the world (materialism). This partial detachment is deemed necessary to prepare for the next life. In this stage, the couples "pay back" to the society by nurturing and grooming the next generation. They spend more time with the young ones (*Brahmacharis*) imparting the necessary knowledge and skills. After having paid back and discharged their responsibilities, the couples literally withdraw, moving away from the society and the material world. This final phase of total renunciation, termed *Sannyasa*, coincides with old age.

OTHER DEVELOPMENTAL THEORIES

A few other developmental theories like Vygotsky's, Bowlby's, and Bronfenbrenner's have clinical relevance in understanding child behavior and counseling techniques.

- *Bowlby's attachment theory* states that children who receive consistent care by a maternal figure or caregiver in the first two years of life build secure attachment.
  Children who have a disorganized or ambivalent or avoidant attachment have difficulty in forming healthy relationships later in childhood and adulthood.
- *Vygotsky's sociocultural theory* states that for learning new tasks, children initially need help or scaffolding from teachers, parents, or peers before they can do the tasks on their own.
  Scaffolding reduces the zone of proximal development and encourages independent performance.
- *Bronfenbrenner's ecological systems* theory mentions that child development and behavior are influenced by complex interaction between multiple systems, namely microsystem (parents, teachers, peers), mesosystem (interpersonal interactions), exosystem (governmental policies, media, community resources),

macrosystem (sociocultural ideologies), and chronosystem (shifts or transitions like parental divorce, wars, climate disasters).

CONCLUSION

Most of the developmental theories talk of expectations—biological, psychological, social, and cultural—that progressively change from one life stage to the next. Such an understanding is important in order to understand the individual presenting herself/himself for counseling. Only by understanding the individual, will one be able to undertake a proper intervention. Furthermore, a good knowledge about various developmental theories raises the possibility of considering an eclectic approach to counseling. Hence, various developmental theories become relevant to the practitioners.

SUGGESTED READING

1. Ashford R, Lecroy E, Jose C. Human Behavior in Social Environment. New York: Brookes and Cole; 1999.
2. Baron RL. Introduction to Psychology. New Delhi: Prentice Hall; 1999.
3. Boeree CG, Buddha SG. In: Baines L, McBrayer D (Eds), How to Get a Life. Lake Worth, FL: Humanics; 2003.
4. Boeree CG. (2003). General Psychology. Jean Piaget and cognitive development. [online] Available from http://webspace.ship.edu/cgboer/genpsypiaget.html [Last accessed August, 2024].
5. Cumming E, Henry WE. Growing Old: The Process of Disengagement. New York: Basic Books; 1961.
6. Devadas R. Child Development. New Delhi: Tata-McGraw Hill; 1981.
7. Erikson Erik H. Childhood and Society. New York: Norton; 1950.
8. Erikson Erik H. Identity and the Life Cycle. New York: International Universities Press; 1959.
9. Estes CL. The social construction of reality: a framework for inquiry. In: Lee PR, Ramsay NB, Red I (Eds). The Nation's Health. San Francisco: Boyd and Fraser; 1981.
10. Fenichel O. An outline of psychoanalysis. Sigmund Freud. Int. J. Psa., XXI, 1940, p. 1. Psychoanal Q. 1941;10:169-73.
11. Hoare CH. Erikson on Development in Adulthood: New Insights from the Unpublished Papers. Oxford: Oxford University Press; 2002.
12. Kohlberg L. The claim to moral adequacy of a highest stage of moral judgment. J Philos. 1973;70:630-46.

13. Macomber LP. Piaget and cognitive development. In: Appel MH, Goldberg L (Eds). Topics in Cognitive Development. New York: Plenum Press; 1997.
14. Main P. (2022). Child development theories. Cognitive development. [online] Available from https://www.structural-learning.com/post/child-development-theories [Last accessed August, 2024].
15. Piaget J. Piaget's theory. In: Mussen P (Ed). Handbook of Child Psychology, 4th edition, vol. 1. New York: Wiley; 1983.
16. Piaget J. Studies in Reflecting Abstraction. Hove, UK: Psychology Press; 2001.
17. Piaget J. The Construction of Reality in the Child. New York: Basic Books; 1954.
18. Roazen P, Erik Erikson H. The Power and Limits of a Vision. New York: The Free Press; 1976.
19. Saunders L. Dorland's Medical Dictionary for Health Consumers. Amsterdam: Elsevier; 2007.
20. Sigmund F. The origin and development of psychoanalysis. Am J Psychol. 1910:21(2):181-218.
21. Zastrow C. Practice of Social Work. New York: Brookes and Cole; 1994.

3 CHAPTER

Adolescent Parenting

Rekha RS, MKC Nair

INTRODUCTION

A person with a poetic disposition would describe adolescence as the most fascinating period of life, full of fun and frolic. But parents who have an adolescent child would probably define it as the most stressful period of parenting life cycle, wherein:

- At one moment, parents feel that children have grown up, and at the next, they realize that they are worse than small kids.
- The period when the adolescents prefer the company of friends or the privacy of their room to spending time with parents
- Complaints of parents intruding in personal matters are common, compounded with the habit of doing things just the opposite of what their parents had wanted.
- Start hanging out late, in spite of parents' advice and threats, either spend too much time in front of the mirror or are extremely careless about dressing, brood over silly matters like pimples and figure, which are of no concern to parents
- Start experimenting with their first smoke and skip meals as they are extremely figure conscious but at the same time have the bad habit of eating out often
- Lot of infatuations, broken hearts are not rare, and they also show emotional liability on the slightest provocation.
- Find it difficult to handle the rapid physiological and associated physical and mental changes
- The children's secretiveness and rebelliousness make it more difficult for them to confide in their parents even if they are good confidantes.

PARENTING ISSUES

Parents are not sure how to tackle their adolescents, and parental efforts to make life with teenagers easy are not always met with success. But that does not mean that the crux of the problem lies with the adolescents themselves. At times, problems occur when parents are unable to grow up with their adolescents. Hence, to make the task for parenting adolescents easier, parents need to understand the peculiarities of this stage and should think of what can be done, what should be done, and what should not be done while their children pass through this challenging period of life.

More Physical Comforts and Loss of Attention

In the olden days, when there were too many children in the family and only limited resources, parents struggled hard to meet the basic needs of children. Hence, yesteryear's children had a goal in life, whether it was good education, a well-paid job, or a decent living, which always kept them going. Nowadays, parents, probably in an effort to give all comforts and luxury that they had been denied in their childhood, are providing more than what is possible for their children and at the same time are brushing aside their children's craving for affection and attention. This can create an increasing feeling of emptiness in children when they have no goals in life and it can also lead to severe interpersonal problems, especially in marriage, as they are unknowingly imbibing the idea that caring is just providing physical comforts and luxuries. Hence, children should not be provided with more than what is needed and, instead, parents should spend more time with them and show their affection through gestures like remembering the children's good deeds, discussing personal problems and family issues, and participating in the parent–teacher meetings.

Role Confusion

For parents, children always remain children and they sometimes tend to treat adolescents as kids. This aggravates the role confusion or dilemma in adolescents as they are treated like adults at one moment and like children at the next. When adolescents take up new roles, it is not uncommon that they err. Instead of finding fault with them, parents should train them to realize where they have gone wrong and to take mistakes in their stride, rather than feeling too much guilty about it.

Low Stress Tolerance

Parents are always there, behind children, telling them what to do and what not to do and if possible doing things which they themselves can manage, whereby they see only the end product and are not aware of the obstacles in achieving the goals, the alternatives available, and how to get things done with patience, perseverance, and endurance. If placed in a difficult situation, these children fall easy prey to it and succumb without even considering the available options. The increase in suicidal rates and depression among teenagers throws light on their very low stress tolerance. Hence, parents should make it a point not to do things for children which they themselves can manage; instead, they should assign small responsibilities to their children and guide them when necessary; this will instill trust and confidence in themselves, so that in future they can safely tide over the times of crisis.

Lack of Access to Information on Healthy Sexuality

It is during this period that they develop interest in the opposite sex. But for parents, it is difficult to come to terms with the fact that their child is grown up enough to have a liking for the opposite sex. Similarly, masturbation is also not uncommon among adolescents, especially boys. Problems due to misconceptions about sex are higher as they lack access to right information on sex and sexuality. Most of the parents, teachers, and elders do not know how to explain sexuality in simple, nonembarrassing words. Parents themselves are shy and secretive about sex. The only available information is from lay magazines online pornography, social media and wrong information passed on by peers, which helps in giving only a distorted idea about sex and sexuality, thereby causing fear, embarrassment, and guilt in adolescents. Parents are aware of the dangers associated with these unscientific sources of sex education, but they do not know how to provide the same.

Period of Value Conflict

Adolescence is a period of value conflict. Adolescents do not know what is right and what is wrong. Hence, during this period, if adolescents do not have a strong value base and willpower, the chances of succumbing to peer pressure and thereby engaging in undesirable acts like smoking, alcoholism, drug addiction, and premarital sex are immense. Hence, parents should try to develop self-love in their children. Self-love does not mean being selfish. If a person loves himself, he will be able to avoid doing things that will prove harmful to him and only such a person can really care for others.

SKILLS NEEDED IN ADOLESCENCE

Adolescence is a period of experimenting, experiencing, and expanding. What parents should do is understand their adolescents, and safeguard, protect, and guide them safely through this period. Adolescents need help and guidance in the following aspects:

- *Decision making:* Remember, to be or not to be is a problem of not just adolescents alone but of adults also.
- *Problem solving:* Here parents have to be extra careful in offering help in solving the problems of adolescents because, although they need help, they are ashamed of acknowledging the fact that they require assistance whereby the chances of aggravating the problem are high.
- *Effective communication:* As adolescents want to be close to their parents and at the same time away from them, they may be rebellious. Here parents should always see to it that they keep the line of communication with their adolescents open.
- *Other skills:* Developing skills in enhancing interpersonal relationship, self-awareness, empathy, coping with stress, and managing emotions are important for adolescents.

All youth need support and guidance. But some young people whose adolescence is marked by more serious struggles may require help from outside the family. Many people believe that family matters should be kept private. Seeking help, however, simply means that the caregiver is drawing on every community resource that can be used to support your child. It is never too late to reach out for help.

DANGER SIGNALS IN ADOLESCENTS

- Large amounts of time spent alone and in isolation from family and friends

- Sudden changes in school performance
- Drastic mood swings or changes in behavior
- Changes in your child's peer group or separation from long-time friends
- Lack of interest in hobbies or social and recreational activities

Keep in mind that these signs do not always mean that the adolescent is in trouble. Some changes in friendships, for example, are normal as young people mature and find new interests. Changes in the family situation, temperamental differences, and sudden crises can trigger off problem behaviors which may be complicated by the normative adolescent behavior of not wanting to share feelings and experiences.

The first step for parents in dealing with concerns about their adolescents, therefore, is to improve or reopen the lines of communication. If problems appear to persist and the child seems reluctant or unable to discuss them, the parent can try talking with him/her in a nonconfrontational manner about the changes noticed. Parents can express their concern for the child's well-being and show interest in helping in any way possible. But they should be prepared for defensive reactions. They should be willing to help their adolescent child and talk through problems, rather than immediately giving solutions.

Parents will be troubled by the confrontational nature of some of the adolescent behavior. It is not an easy job to decide where you should draw the limits and where you should give in. Hence, there is no tailor-made solutions to these problems. Each of us develops our own strategies in dealing with our adolescents at times through trial and error, through experience and at times adopting the practices which our parents had followed with us. But certain strategies that would certainly help in the understanding and handling of adolescents are as follows:

- Parents should try to be good role models.
- Try to keep the communication alive, especially between mothers and daughters, and thereby create a feeling that I am here for you.
- Parents should take efforts to understand adolescent development. Learn about the behaviors to expect, the effects of

physical changes, and the ways to help the teenager to deal with change.

- Help to choose good friends before friendship is established.
- Provide right information on sex and sexuality, without creating anxiety in them.
- Encourage developing sharing, good habits, and autonomy, and instill in them a good value system.
- Give them freedom but within limits.
- Avoid unhealthy comparisons and cursing adolescents.
- Be authoritative and not authoritarian (autocrat).
- Instill confidence and trust in adolescents.
- Help to keep body and mind clean and healthy through yoga, social service, National Service Scheme (NSS), and spiritual activities. This helps not only to channelize extra energy but also to develop confidence.

ADOLESCENT PARENTING: TIPS

- Educate yourself about adolescent development. Learn about the behaviors to be expected, the effects of physical changes, and the ways to help your child deal with change.
- Remember your own adolescence. Remember your own changing feelings, anger at authority, fears, and hopes. Look at your adolescent's behavior in the context of those memories to help you keep perspective.
- Parenting is a learned skill. Training can help even experienced parents by giving them new tools for supporting children through adolescence. Talking to other parents about their own experiences in handling adolescent children can be very helpful.
- Listen more than talking. Young people have spent at least a decade as listeners in most situations. During adolescence, they want to and need the chance to share their feelings and ideas and to begin recasting family beliefs, stories, and traditions in the light of their changing identity.
- Teach adolescents about the joys and the troubles in life and ways to revel in the good times and cope with the bad. The myth that life is always easy or fair or that one should always be happy can lead to frustration for young people facing the realities of life.

- Use positive reinforcement for positive behavior whenever possible; it is far more effective than criticism or punishment for negative behavior. Words that belittle can hurt an adolescent's self-esteem. The most useful tools in raising young people are sensitivity, praise, understanding, and communication.
- Teach adolescents that rights and responsibilities go hand in hand and give the child increasing responsibility for his/her personal well-being and that of the family. Provide the child opportunities to help around the house and to become involved in decision-making discussions in the family. In doing so, seeking the child's input enables him/her to understand the processes that can be used in making those decisions.
- Look for situations that can allow a child to test decision-making skills with the support of caring adults. Supportive adults can help provide the child with an understanding of the impact of those decisions on both the child and the others. They also can assist the adolescent in coping with the results of these choices.
- Helping an adolescent to move toward independence is a key thing. For every youth, the need to assert independence will happen at different times and through different means. Becoming attuned to children's attempts to operate independently will help in supporting those efforts and providing guidance when early attempts at decision-result in less-than-desired outcomes. It is sometimes difficult for parents to give up control out of concern for their child's safety. Adolescents' skills in coping with increasing responsibility will be enhanced by parents' willingness to support them as they make choices and face new challenges.
- Offer the child chances to become involved in the community. All young people are searching for their place in the world. Involving adolescents in developing solutions to community problems can shift their focus from themselves and help them to develop skills and feel involved and empowered.
- Spend quality and quantity time with adolescents. Adolescence is a time when young people naturally begin to pull away from the family and spend more time at school, with friends, or at a job. Still, the time spent with caring parents is key to young people's

ability to grow emotionally and socially. Take advantage of times that the adolescent is home, over dinner or watching a cricket match, to continue building your relationship.

- Getting involved in the child's outdoor interests can be useful. A sincere attempt at involvement will both convince the child of your support and help the parents to remain informed about the child's interests.
- Treating your adolescent child's friends with respect and care is a must for him/her to accept you as a responsible parent and not just an adult tyrant.
- Parents have to accept that the adolescents too have feelings. Parents may feel frustrated, angry, discouraged, or sad during difficult times with their adolescent. Being a good parent does not mean being perfect. Modeling the ability to apologize when parents have an inappropriate showdown with their children or others will set an example and help the child to understand the human frailty. It will also teach them ways to mend relationships strained by stress or disagreement.
- Seeking support and guidance for the parent in dealing with the changes in a child moving through adolescence may also be needed. Learn about the signs of crisis and talk with other parents or professionals. By doing so, the parent can begin to tell the difference between adolescent behavior that indicates a youth in crisis and the usual behavior associated with a life passage.
- Remember that most youth have problems at some time or other. Acting-out behavior can be a normal part of becoming an adult. Parents sometimes needlessly feel embarrassed when their children are having trouble. A parent need not assume that the child's behavior always reflects on the quality of his/her parenting.
- Do not always push for drastic or dramatic solutions. Sometimes, young people just need time and support to work through their problems.
- Parents should never attempt to foist their unrealized academic and career dreams on their offspring. This becomes all the more unrealistic and potentially risky when the youngster has little interest or aptitude for the parental choices.

- Digital parenting is essential in the current era of media boom. Parents need to role-model mindful media use. They should mentor their children regarding advantages and hazards of media use and online etiquette and encourage them to be a responsible digital citizen. Parents need to update themselves regarding the latest digital innovations like artificial intelligence, closely monitor the online lives of their children, set limits and boundaries, and keep the channels of communication open to navigate risks like cyberbullying and online sexual solicitation. They should ensure that recreational screen time should not interfere with scholastic pursuits, exercise, hobbies, in-person family interactions, and sleep. Digital fasting days/schedule and media-free zones (kitchen, bedroom, car, dining table) should be specified by the parents to reduce screen usage.

CONCLUSION

Parents should provide children with positive feedback and opportunities to grow and reflect in adolescence. Health, happiness, movement toward a promising future, and offering them chances to strengthen their skills and develop a sense of competence, usefulness, and belonging constitutes the matrix of parenting an adolescent.

SUGGESTED READING

1. Galagali P. Adolescent Parenting in IAP Child Care: A Parents' Manual. Ed: Abraham Paul. Pee Pee Publishers 2016. pp. 344-51.
2. Gupta P, Shah D, Bedi N, Galagali P, Dalwai S, Agrawal S, et al. Indian Academy of Pediatrics guidelines on screen time and digital wellness in infants, children and adolescents. Indian Pediatr. 2022;59:235-44.
3. Teens: Behaviour. Raising Children.net.au: the Australian parenting website. Accessed on 10 December 2024 https://raisingchildren.net.au/teens/behaviour
4. Yamuna S, Vijayarani M. Parenting an Adolescent. In Adolescent Friendly Pediatric Practice. Ed: Pemde H, Ratna Kumari TL, Galagali PM, Velmurugan. Jaypee Bros Medical Publishers Pvt Limited 2024. pp. 43-9.

4 CHAPTER

Adolescent Sexuality

MKC Nair, Resmi VR

INTRODUCTION

Sexuality is a boon given to mankind by the Almighty. It is the sum total of one's thinking, behavior, and attitude. Sexuality is becoming comfortable with one's own body, emotions, and feelings. To develop a positive sexuality concept, one has to free the mind from all the fears, misconceptions, myths, and complexes.

A decade ago, it was considered taboo to talk about sex. But the emergence of sexually transmitted infections (STI) and human immunodeficiency virus (HIV)/acquired immunodeficiency syndrome (AIDS) has renewed interest in this subject. Child prostitution is now considered a social menace. Sexual abuse of children is now increasingly being recognized, creating further parental anxiety. Many wonder whether sexual freedom is responsible for the increasing number of unwanted teenage pregnancy. In 1997, the Reproductive and Child Health (RCH) program of the Government of India implemented under the National Rural Health Mission (NRHM) gave us an opportunity for the first time to plan and execute concrete actions for promoting adolescent reproductive health. However, many of us are not yet ready to accept sex education for our children in school and hence a more acceptable term "family life education" is now being used. The Indian Academy of Pediatrics (IAP) has committed itself for promoting the cause of adolescents with the slogan *"We promise to look after you, till you are 18".*

EVOLVING HEALTHY SEXUALITY

This has to be a lifelong process and should start at infancy itself, something that most parents do not realize. For example, when the mother is giving bath to the baby, she talks about the head, nose, mouth, arms, and tummy and then goes on to the legs skipping the genitals, leaving a lifelong doubt and confusion in the mind of the child.

The 3- to 6-year-old (phallic stage) would be handling the genitals, which is only part of the normal sexual identification as male and female. But the parents equate it with adult sexual behavior, scold him/her for nothing, and produce lifelong guilt feeling in the child.

Every adolescent has to be prepared for evolving healthy sexuality, by promoting good interpersonal relationship, with confidence to face a person of the opposite sex. Every girl has to be made aware that sexual relations are also like any other human relations, to be learned and to be evolved over time. Societal and family values and good upbringing with the father as the role model help the adolescent boy to become comfortable with his own sex and sexuality as well as learn to respect a woman as a human being having a mind of her own. But the process is not easy as the adolescents are in dilemma, as they do not understand their body, cannot accept their body image, and keep on worrying how to make themselves more appealing.

Adolescence is characterized by three "E's"—experimenting, experiencing, and expanding—the adolescents' effort to come to terms with their own sexual feelings and establishing a positive sexual identity. Sexual identity has different dimensions:

- Physical
- Psychological
- Sociocultural
- Spiritual
- Esthetic
- Romantic
- Existential

Sexuality indeed is a gestalt or unique integration of all these.

SEXUALITY PROBLEMS IN ADOLESCENCE

Adolescents do have sexuality-related problems and many factors have been identified to be related to them:

- Nonavailability of proper scientific information and guidance

- Incapacity of parents, elders, and teachers to impart information in a natural way
- Distorted ideas among peers sharing online pornographic material and unscientific lay magazines
- Fear, embarrassment, and guilt to express themselves
- Alcoholic father—lack of warmth in family relations
- Pathological families—uninhibited sexual behavior of the father
- Tying adolescents to parent's 'apron strings", even after they are grown up
- Parents being unduly shy and secretive with a lot of taboos and prohibitions
- Sex abuse—fear of the unknown

The print, digital and social media, television, and films have all influenced the sexuality concepts of youngsters. Media have often projected the female sex more as an instrument for enjoyment, an object for deriving pleasure, and a sales promotion tool. Although interest in nudity is only a healthy expression of adolescent curiosity, getting hooked to blue films at this age may distort the image of a woman from being a mother, wife, sister, or daughter to only a sex toy to be used and misused, just for one's own pleasure and at will.

The initial expressions of an adolescent girl's sexuality may be related to her acceptance of the process of menstruation. The onset of menstruation (menarche) may be an unpleasant, sometimes frightening experience for an uninformed girl. The common menstrual problems of pain accompanying the onset of flow and vaginal discharge and discomfort may prevent her from accepting menses as a "welcome nuisance". While the girls are concerned with excessive hair growth on the body, the boys may be concerned about the lack of it. While the girls are concerned about the small size of the breasts, the boys may be embarrassed by the excess growth of them (gynecomastia). While the boys are eagerly awaiting an opportunity to prove their sexual powers, the girls may be concerned with keeping their virginity intact and have underlying fears about unwanted pregnancy.

Just as onset of menses denotes sexual maturity in girls, wet dreams denote the onset of sexual maturity among boys.

Whereas the age of sexual maturity for boys is reached by 13 years, the opportunity for marital sexual relations does not usually come before the age of 25 years, a clear gap of 12 years, necessitating other outlets; the least harmful among them is masturbation [World Health Organization (WHO)]. Masturbation among boys is a universal phenomenon, whereas in girls, it may not be so and hence it may be more appropriate to present it as "not abnormal." Traditionally, masturbation being a taboo subject may provoke intense feeling of guilt and fears of becoming impotent, causing blurring of eyesight, diminishing size of the penis, weakness, health hazards, loss of intellectual ability, and even possible insanity. The sexuality counseling at this age should be directed toward removing these unfounded fears.

This also involves improving the self-esteem of the person, through proper scientific explanations and reassurance that masturbation is a universal biological phenomenon with no harm to the body or mind, unless obsessed with it to the extent that the routines are disturbed. Such a person should be helped to develop more socialization by indulging in socially acceptable companionships. It may be most disturbing to the child if the parents, particularly the mother, come to know about it. In young children, most often the initiation of masturbation-like actions is by local irritation or repeated rubbing of genitals done unknowingly by parents while bathing, leading to arousal even at a young age.

Homosexuality at this age may often be only a homosocial behavior, a passing phase, an outlet for sexual urge coupled with lack of heterosexual outlet.

Gender is a social construct and it is the internal feeling of being a boy or a girl. Gender identity is established usually in childhood and finally emerges as a sense of self in adolescence and youth. An individual is cis-gender when the gender identity is similar to the sex assigned at birth and gender nonconforming or transgender when it is not similar to it. Transgenders may face stigmatization, abuse, mental distress, and gender dysphoria. Counseling regarding healthy sexual relationships and gender-affirming care should be imparted with a nonjudgmental empathetic attitude.

SEXUAL RELATIONSHIPS

- These should never be coercive or exploitive. Such relationships bring sexual pleasure to one person at the expense of the other. This degrades the latter's human dignity and self-worth.
- These should be based on mutual trust, honesty, commitment, and respect. These should be one of sharing, caring, and loving on both sides.
- These should be gender sensitive. To achieve this, all children should be loved and cared for. Both male and female children should be treated equally, since both of them grow up to take part in procreation. Men and women are an integral part of society and, hence, both should be treated alike right from their birth.
- All sexual decisions have effects or consequences. These effects may be positive or negative, immediate or long term.
- All persons have the right and the obligation to make responsible sexual choices. Every individual has the right to make decisions, which bring him/her personal happiness. At the same time, each person has the responsibility to ensure that these choices do not deprive other people of their happiness.
- Individuals and society benefit when children are able to discuss sexuality with their parents and/or with other trusted adults.
- Young people explore their sexuality as a natural process of achieving sexual maturity.
- Premature involvement in sexual behavior poses risks.
- Sexual behavior must be responsible and self-disciplined.
- For adolescents, abstaining from sexual intercourse (abstinence) is the most effective method of avoiding pregnancy and preventing sexually transmitted diseases (STDs) and HIV/AIDS.
- Young people who are involved in sexual relationships need access to information about healthcare services.

SEX AND SEXUALITY SESSIONS

Objectives

After attending such a session, the participants should be able to understand:

- What human sexuality is
- The functions of the sex organs

- Normal development and variations during puberty
- Myths and facts about sex and sexuality
- Ability to accept own sexual feelings and needs
- Acceptance that differences exist among people

Methods

- Participants to think of puberty changes
- Participants to name one change in them
- Write same under different headings (physical, emotional, mental, and social)
- Emphasize that all are equally important
- Define human sexuality
- Describe all possible variations—all dimensions

Introducing Embarrassing Words

Participant embarrassment is normal, but the faculty has to be comfortable with the topic.

- *Masturbation (self-stimulation):* Say not abnormal—if you say abnormal, it provokes guilt in those who are indulging in it, and if you say normal, you may be perceived as promoting it. In a lighter vein, you could say, "*You have a right to scratch any part of your body, but do not overdo it and make it an ulcer!!!" (Children enjoy it).*
- *Sexual intercourse in marriage:* Mutual surrender of mind, body, and soul for mutual pleasure/orgasm (physical), ecstasy (mental), and fulfillment (spiritual).
- *Rape:* A brutal invasion of your privacy, not only of the body but also of the mind.
- *Homosexuality/lesbianism:* Considered only a different sexual orientation.

MYTHS AND MISCONCEPTIONS

Knowledge regarding sex and sexuality is acquired through various formal and informal means. Much of the information acquired through informal sources is unlikely to be accurate or correct. Sex being a topic that is not openly discussed, many myths and misconceptions circulate in society. These myths can be wiped out only by providing accurate scientific information through effective sexuality education programs. Some of the common myths and misconceptions in our society are listed as follows:

- Education in human sexuality in schools and colleges will lead to sexual experimentation—*false.*
- One drop of semen is equivalent to 40 drops of blood, which in turn requires a lot of nourishing food—*false.*
- Nocturnal emissions or wet dreams indicate a sexual disorder—*false.*
- The presence of a hymen is the only test of a woman's virginity—*false.*
- Larger breasts produce more milk than smaller ones—*false.*
- A woman is impure during menstruation—*false.*
- Menopause is the end of sex life—*false.*
- Sexual intercourse should be avoided during menses—*false.*
- Sterilization reduces sexual desire and capacity of men and women—*false.*
- Masturbation is practiced exclusively by men and can lead to insanity, impotence, homosexuality, dark circles around the eyes, mental retardation, diminishing size of the penis, and changes in the angle of the penis—*false.*
- Homosexuals can be identified by their appearance—*false.*
- If a man with a STI has sex with a virgin girl, he will be cured of the STDs—*false.*
- HIV-positive persons can be identified by their appearance—*false.*
- A large penis is of greater importance to a woman's sexual gratification—*false.*

SEXUALITY: THE SUM TOTAL

- *The physical:* To enjoy beauty is not a sin—humans are the best creations of God.
- *The mental:* "Giving type"—contentment in making the partner happy and give pleasure (orgasm), with an umpteen number of opportunities and ways to experiment. It is likely that your partner would return the favors with compound interest. You will not have to look outside your home for pleasure opportunities.
- *The spiritual:* Do not hurt others if possible and do not hurt yourself ever.

Oath: I am the custodian of my mind, body and spirit; I will protect, preserve and enhance it.

—*MKC Nair*

CONCLUSION

Sexuality is a complex idea that involves physical make-up, how one thinks and feels about himself/herself, other people and the society and thereby behaves with them. It is influenced by biological, social, psychological, digital, spiritual, religious, political, legal, historical, ethical and cultural factors. Sexuality includes body image, gender identity, gender roles, gender expression, sexual orientation, pleasure, intimacy, personal values, sex and reproduction. Sexuality develops, evolves and changes over the life span and is an important determinant of overall well-being of an individual. In our society, speaking about sexuality is considered a taboo and an open dialogue or conversation with children and adolescents is discouraged. Comprehensive sexuality education program is a science, curriculum and rights based, process of learning and teaching that is age, developmentally and culturally appropriate. It aims to foster affirmative sexuality and enable individuals to nurture happy, safe, healthy and responsible sexual behavior and relationships that are free from coercion and violence. Research has shown that in adolescents who receive sexuality education, there is a delay in initiation of sexual activity, decrease in the frequency of sexual intercourse, in the number of sexual partners and in risky sexual behaviors.

SUGGESTED READING

1. Goldfarb ES, Lieberman LD. Three Decades of Research: The Case for Comprehensive Sex Education. J Adolesc Health. 2021;68:13-27.
2. Herat J, Plesons M, Castle C, et al. The revised international technical guidance on sexuality education—a powerful tool at an important crossroads for sexuality education. Reprod Health. 2018;15(1):185.
3. Pemde HK, Bansal U, Bhattacharya P, Sharma RN, Kumar S, Bhatia P, et al. Adolescent Health Academy statement on the care of transgender children, adolescents, and youth. Indian Pediatr. 2023;60:843-54.

5 CHAPTER

Adolescent Behavior Problems

Anil Kumar TV, Indu PS

INTRODUCTION

The current understanding of behavioral problems is that they result from interplay between biological (brain neurotransmitters), psychological (personality), and social (family, environment) factors. This approach is a more objective view and helps us analyze the problems more clearly and plan effective treatment. For example, at the intervention level, we have drugs at the biological domain, psychotherapy at the psychological domain, and family therapy and environmental modification at the social domain. Failure of early identification and timely intervention can affect the adolescent and the family in a major way.

Although common, many of the behavioral problems noted in adolescence are taken as part of normal "adolescent blues". This chapter is based on the experience of conducting Child Guidance Clinic at SAT Hospital, Medical College, Thiruvananthapuram.

The common mental health issues seen in adolescents include scholastic backwardness, family conflicts, intellectual and learning disabilities, attention-deficit hyperactivity disorder (ADHD), somatoform disorders, oppositional defiant disorder, speech problems, stammering, fear, anxiety, separation anxiety and school phobia.

In the Child and Adolescent Psychiatry Clinic at Medical College, Thiruvananthapuram, Kerala, India, the following problems were seen, listed in the order of their frequency:

- Conduct disorder
- Depression
- Conversion disorder
- Adjustment disorder

- Hyperactivity
- Mania
- Anxiety disorder
- Psychosis
- *Others:* Tic disorders, enuresis, post-traumatic stress disorder (PTSD), behavior problems due to general medical condition [e.g., encephalitis, systemic lupus erythematosus (SLE)]
- *Special problems:* Substance abuse—alcohol, nicotine, opioids (commonly seen in conduct disorder, ADHD); suicide attempt (seen in depression, personality disorder)

AGGRESSIVE CHILD

Conduct Disorder

Conduct disorder is characterized by a repetitive and persistent pattern of anti-social, aggressive, or defiant conduct. The diagnostic features are excessive levels of fighting or bullying, cruelty to animals and other people, severe destruction to property, fire setting, stealing, repeated lying, truancy from school, running away from home, unusually frequent and severe temper tantrums, defiant provocative behavior, and persistent severe disobedience.

The above symptoms should be present for >6 months to make a diagnosis of conduct disorder. At the same time, comorbidity is common in conduct disorder. We should look for comorbid conditions, such as substance use, hyperactivity, and depression, in all cases of conduct disorder.

Nonpharmacological intervention is the mainstay of treatment in conduct disorder. This includes individual and family therapy. The indications for drug treatment are comorbidity, failure of nonpharmacological intervention, and severe symptoms. The drugs used are clonidine, risperidone, and carbamazepine.

DEPRESSED CHILD

Depression

At any point of time, depression is seen in about 5% of children and adolescents. To make the diagnosis of depression, persistence of sadness of mood or decreased interest in daily activities should be present for >2 weeks, along with four of the following symptoms:

1. Disturbed sleep
2. Change in appetite
3. Expressing hopelessness, worthlessness
4. Thoughts or expressions of suicide
5. Complaints of decreased energy; frequent complaints of headache, body pain, etc.
6. Psychomotor retardation (e.g., withdrawal from friends)
7. Complaining of memory impairment and decreased concentration (e.g., poor academic performance).

Depression can be managed with drug treatment (antidepressants, e.g., fluoxetine, sertraline) for 6 months to 1 year, along with psychosocial support. Recurrent depression warrants prolonged drug treatment. If there is a history of a manic episode, mood stabilizers are indicated.

The situations in which the adolescent child has to be referred to a psychiatrist are failure of response to drugs, deterioration of symptoms, increased or new suicidal thoughts, frequent relapses, atypical symptoms, psychotic symptoms, and presence of substance abuse.

FUNCTIONAL CHILD

Somatoform Disorder

The term hysteria should be avoided and the most common somatoform disorder, previously called conversion problem, seen in the clinic is pseudoseizure. It is extremely difficult to resolve some cases of pseudoseizures. During evaluation, one has to look for the classical features of true seizures, comorbid conditions (depression should not be missed in pseudoseizures), and any psychological stressor. Management includes measures to counter the illness behavior and sick role of the child. Individual psychotherapy will help to elicit the stress, resolve the conflict, and improve the coping skills. Family education and counseling will also help in managing somatoform disorder.

CHILD IN DISTRESS

Adjustment Disorder

Behavior problems can arise during a period requiring adaptation to a significant life change or to a stressful life event (e.g., physical illness, bereavement, migration). The clinical features include depressed mood, anxiety, and worries. Treatment is mainly nonpharmacological, such as psychosocial intervention.

INATTENTIVE CHILD

Attention-deficit/Hyperactivity Disorder

The cardinal features are impaired attention and overactivity. They usually present with problems in studies. Comorbid learning disability and conduct disorder are very common. The nonpharmacological treatment includes behavior therapy, parent training, and special attention given to the child at school. Drugs such as stimulants (e.g., methylphenidate), atomoxetine, and clonidine also help in managing ADHD.

GRANDIOSE REBELLIOUS CHILD

Mania

Mania is an episodic illness, with a definite change in behavior, different from the previous pattern. The diagnosis of mania can be made if the mood is persistently elated or irritable for at least 1 week, with three of the following symptoms:

1. Increased self-esteem
2. Sleep disturbance
3. Distractibility
4. Psychomotor overactivity
5. Excessive talk
6. Flight of ideas
7. Increased indulgence in pleasurable activities, such as smoking, alcohol use, hypersexual behavior.

Mood stabilizers (e.g., lithium, sodium valproate, carbamazepine) form the sheet anchor of treatment of mania. They have a prophylactic role in preventing further episodes.

ANXIOUS CHILD

Anxiety and Obsessive–Compulsive Disorders

Anxiety disorders include generalized anxiety disorder, phobias (social and specific phobia), panic disorder (episodic severe anxiety), social anxiety disorder, separation anxiety disorder, and selective mutism. Obsessive-compulsive and related disorders include obsessive-compulsive disorder (OCD), body dysmorphic disorder, trichotillomania, skin picking disorder, etc. Depending on the severity of individual problems, pharmacological and nonpharmacological measures are needed. Individual psychotherapy/behavior therapy may help. The drugs used are benzodiazepines on a short term basis to relieve anxious feelings and antidepressants for 6–9 months usually.

CHILD WITH ODD THINKING AND ODD BEHAVIOR

Psychosis–Schizophrenia

The term psychosis is used only when delusions and hallucinations are present. The reality orientation is lost (not delirium!). Schizophrenia is a serious mental illness and the most disabling illness in this age group. Early diagnosis and initiation of drug treatment are essential to prevent chronic disability. Two out of five of the following criteria should be present, for 1 month, to diagnose schizophrenia:

1. Delusions (firmly held ideas that are plainly false and not shared by others in the person's social group)
2. Hallucinations (false or imaginary sensation, e.g., hearing voices)
3. Disorganized speech (incoherent speech)
4. Disorganized or catatonic features (e.g., posturing, mutism)
5. Negative symptoms (e.g., severe social withdrawal).

Pharmacological intervention is "the treatment of choice" in schizophrenia. The antipsychotics include conventional drugs like haloperidol and newer ones such as risperidone, olanzapine, and clozapine **(Table 1)**. The World Health Organization recommends a psychiatry consultation for all "new" cases of psychosis.

Psychopharmacology in a nutshell for psychiatrist is given in **Table 1**.

TABLE 1: Commonly used drugs in child and adolescent psychiatry.

Drug	*Starting dose*	*Usual daily dose*
Antidepressants		
Fluoxetine (cap. 20 mg)	*Children and teens:* 5 mg	*Children and teens:* 20 mg
Liquid (20 mg/5 mL)	*Children:* 25 mg	*Children and teens:* 50 mg
Sertraline (tab. 50 mg)	*Teens:* 50 mg	
Antipsychotics		
Haloperidol (tab. 1.5, 5, 10 mg; inj. 5 mg/mL; liquid 2 mg/mL)	1 mg	5–15 mg
Risperidone (tab. 1, 2, 3 mg; liquid 1 mg/mL)	0.5 mg	2–6 mg
Mood stabilizers		
Lithium (tab. 300, 400 mg)	*Children:* 150 mg	*Children:* 600 mg
	Teens: 300 mg	*Teens:* 900 mg (25–30 mg/kg; serum level 0.8–1.2 mEq/L)
Sodium valproate (tab. 200, 300, 500 mg)	*Children:* 125 mg	*Children:* 1,000–1,200 mg
	Teens: 250 mg	*Teens:* 1,000–2,500 mg (30–60 mg/kg)
Others		
Methylphenidate (tab. 10 mg)	5 mg	15–60 mg (0.4–0.8 mg/kg/dose)
Clonidine (tab. 0.1 mg)	0.05 mg	0.1–0.3 mg (4–7 mg/kg)

CONCLUSION

In all cases of adolescents presenting with behavior issues, it is essential to rule out a neurodevelopmental and/or a mental disorder. A referral to a mental health professional is required in cases with severe mental disorder, poor response to counseling for 6 weeks, psychosis, severe substance use disorder, suicidal behavior and post traumatic disorder following childhood trauma.

SUGGESTED READING

1. American Academy of Child and Adolescent Psychiatry. Practice parameters for the assessment and treatment of children and adolescents. Am Acad Child Adolesc Psychiatry. 1997;36(10):122S-39S.
2. American Psychiatric Association. Diagnostic and Statistical Manual of Mental Illness, 5th edition. Washington, DC: American Psychiatric Association; 2013.
3. Green J, Jacobs B (Eds). Patient Child Psychiatry—Modern Practice, Research and the Future. London/New York: Routledge; 1998.
4. Kutcher SP. Child and Adolescent Psychopharmacology. Philadelphia: WB Saunders Company; 1997.
5. Malhotra S. Child Psychiatry in India. An Approach to Assessment and Management of Childhood Psychiatric Disorders. Noida: Macmillan India Ltd; 2002.
6. World Health Organization. (2019/2021). International Classification of Diseases, 11th Revision (ICD-11). Geneva: World Health Organization. [online] Available from https://icd.who.int/browse11 [Last accessed September, 2024].

6 CHAPTER

Ten Good Reasons for Adolescent Counseling

MKC Nair, Paul Swamidhas Sudhakar Russell

INTRODUCTION

In the current era, there is a felt need for adolescent counselling by parents, teachers and adolescents themselves. Adolescents are in a transitional phase of life between childhood and adulthood. It is a period of great opportunity where the adolescent can be counseled and motivated to adopt a healthy lifestyle and coping strategies to overcome life challenges. Ten important reasons for adolescent counseling are discussed in this chapter.

ADOLESCENT PROBLEMS DO HAVE ANTECEDENTS

Majority of our adolescents would be in school and the system is happy with a child who sits quietly and learns things, does homework daily, counts numbers 1–100, reads words, and writes alphabets. Majority of the children would have no problem in following this school routine. But some would have problems from the preschool stage itself, causing difficulties in school and at home, and this is the most commonly observed antecedent for later-on scholastic or school-related problems. What about the learning skills to express oneself and communicate to others? The present-day preschool education focuses on the three R's, and not on providing prereading, prewriting, and prearithmetic skills necessary for formal school education.

Learning in the Preschool Child has Many Dimensions

- *Knowledge:* Preschoolers do not acquire knowledge by reading unlike older ones.
- *Skills:* Skills are learned from direct instruction and improved with practice and drill.

- *Feelings:* Feelings of competence, belonging, and security are acquired.
- *Dispositions:* Curiosity, friendliness, creativity, bossism, etc., are sets of dispositions.

Intellectual Subnormality in Primary Schoolchildren

The primary school age between 6 and 10 years is developmentally the ideal stage for imparting formal education. Most of the innovations in primary education like District Primary Education Programme (DPEP) have focused more on the teaching methods and school infrastructure development. But there is a third dimension to the problem of poor performance in primary classes—intellectual disability. Nair MKC et al., studies have shown that 10% of primary schoolchildren in the government sector in Kerala do have intellectual sub normality and 3% intellectual abnormality.

DEVELOPMENTAL PROBLEMS ARE NOT UNCOMMON

Every child has a right to normal growth and development and we need to ensure this by developmental assessment in the first few years of life. Nair MKC et al., studies using simple tools like Trivandrum Developmental Screening Chart (TDSC) have shown that 2.5% of under-2 children have developmental delay. Attention-deficit/hyperactivity disorder (ADHD) with or without intellectual disability does affect the performance of the primary schoolchildren.

Attention-deficit/hyperactivity disorder is characterized by:
- Symptoms of attention deficit
- Symptoms of hyperactivity/impulsivity
- Present in two or more settings
- Onset before 12 years
- Duration >6 months

*Intellectual disability is characterized by low intelligence coupled with poor social adaptive functions. It is graded according to the intelligence quotient (IQ) level **(Table 1)**.*

TABLE 1: Grading of intellectual disability.

IQ	***Severity abilities***	
70–90	Borderline	Low achievers, educable
70–51	Mild	Educable to certain extent
50–36	Moderate	Self-help skills, trainable
35–21	Severe	Trainable (daycare centers)
0–20	Profound	May need institutional care

(IQ: intelligence quotient)

The problem is compounded by an apparent increase in the number of children with autism spectrum disorders (ASDs), first identified in the toddler stage.

Autism spectrum disorders are characterized by:

- Difficulties in social emotional reciprocity
- Difficulties in nonverbal communication used for social interaction
- Deficits in developing and maintaining relationships
- Restricted-repetitive behavior
- Symptoms must be present in early childhood but may not become fully manifest until social demands exceed limited capacities. Onset is usually before 3 years.

Hypoxic-Ischemic Encephalopathy Severity and Intelligence Quotient at 12 Years

Majority of the babies who have had delay in the first cry (birth asphyxia) do recover soon but those who develop initial symptoms of brain irritation followed by respiratory depression, inability to feed, and repeated convulsions may have hypoxic ischemic encephalopathy (HIE) long-term intellectual consequences. Nair MKC et al., studies have shown that 13% of babies with HIE who were followed up at the age of 12 years had intellectual disability, 56% had borderline and low average intelligence, and only 31% had average and above average intelligence.

Low-birth-weight Babies may have Poor Performance Later in Life

Nearly one-third of babies born in India have birth weight <2,500 g and they are a significant identifiable group with long-term poor intellectual performance. Nair MKC et al., studies have shown that among graduates of neonatal nursery with various medical complications, tested at 13 years of age, 52% of low-birth-weight (LBW)-born group had poor performance as compared with only 42% of normal-birth-weight group.

THERE IS A HUGE DEMAND FOR ADOLESCENT COUNSELING SERVICES

Counseling is required for those adolescents who have scholastic backwardness, adjustment difficulties, character–personality disorders, and specific behavioral problems as well as for non-assertive adolescents. Counseling is not advising, does not solve all life's problems, is aimed at helping people make choices and act on them, is a learning process, and enables personality development. There are many approaches to counseling commonly used:

- *Cognitive approach (cognition means knowing):* The process of counseling is replacing unreasonable thoughts by reasonable ones, i.e., to help clients eliminate most emotional disturbances by learning to think rationally and to help them get rid of illogical, irrational ideas and attitudes and substitute logical rational ideas and attitudes.
- *Affective approach (affect means feeling):* This approach focuses attention on what is going on inside the individual and particularly what he/she is experiencing at a given time. The best example would be the client-centered approach of Rogers, focusing on elimination of defense mechanisms developed out of perception of threat, insecurity, inadequacy, and worthlessness.
- *Behavior approach (conation means doing):* This approach is characterized by a focus on overt and specified behavior, precise and well-spelt-out target behaviors called goals, formulation of a specific and objective treatment procedure to the problem at hand, and an objective assessment of the outcome of counseling in terms of the degree of approximation to the target behavior.

SCHOOL COUNSELING NEEDS HAVE CHANGED OVER THE YEARS

The concept, meaning, and relevance of counseling have changed over the years. In the 1940s, public school teachers' perception of top disciplinary problems in the United States was talking out of turn, chewing gum, making noise, running in halls, cutting in line, dress-code violations, littering, etc., whereas in the 1990s, it had changed to more serious issues like drug abuse, alcohol abuse, rape, teenage pregnancy, suicide, robbery, and assault, and in the 2000s, media-related issues like internet gaming disorder, problematic internet use, cyberbullying, sexting, and nomophobia have gained prominence.

Studies by Nair MKC et al., among class 11 and 12 students of 102 higher secondary schools in Thiruvananthapuram district, using Teenage Screening Questionnaire (TSQ) have shown that 61% had scholastic problems, 32% personal problems, 22% family problems, and 15% adjustment problems.

"THE SPARK FROM WITHIN" NEEDS TO BE IGNITED IN THE ADOLESCENT

We have been teaching many subjects in the school but not how to learn. Children's learning or understanding styles vary and hence the teaching process should facilitate learning in all the three types:

1. Visual learners (learn better by reading line by line/word by word)
2. Auditory learners (learn better by reading aloud)
3. Experiential learners (learn better by experiencing/experimenting).

Studies by Nair MKC et al., have shown that improving the study habits would bring about improvement in academic performance. So, the natural question would be "how to promote good study habits".

- *Have regular study pattern:* Read tomorrow's topic once today, read daily lessons once, and revise in the weekends.
- *Better concentration:* Write down key points and repeat them many times.
- *Reduce personal factors/distractions in studies:* Set targets and insist on meeting the targets. You cannot wish away distractions.
- *Promote ambition and motivation:* Internal (from within) and external (enabling environment).

Most students would complain that they cannot remember the lessons during the examination. We need to understand the fact that at birth, the neuronal connections are thin, but by about 2 years, connections become very dense. Repeated reading improves the neuronal connections and hence recalling becomes very easy. The internet site that you have searched previously would be much easier to access as compared with a new site.

Tips for Improving Memory

- Make associations—mnemonic
- Make key points
- Graphic representations
- Connect related topics and read
- Combined study
- Teach someone else the same topic.

ANXIETY AND STRESS HAVE A HIGH TOLL ON PHYSICAL AND MENTAL WELL-BEING

Anxiety and stress are part of our lives and to some extent help better achievement. But the anxiety curve is curvilinear and beyond a point, it in fact reduces performance. Anxiety disorders (neurotic, stress-related, and somatoform disorders) may include phobic anxiety and other disorders, anxiety, obsessive-compulsive disorders, reaction to severe stress, and adjustment disorders. Many such children may have somatization symptoms like headaches, abdominal distress, neurological disorders—double vision and incoordination, paralysis, seizures, imagined physical deformities or defects, back pain, fatigue, and sore muscles. Post-traumatic stress syndrome is characterized by catastrophic trauma, intrusive recollection, avoidance, and autonomic arousal.

How to Reduce Examination Anxiety?

- Encourage to express difficulties, anxieties, stress factor, and adjustment problems.
- Avoid outside food; have regular home-made food and adequate water intake.

- Regular sleep for a minimum of 7 hours is a must.
- No stimulant to keep awake should be used, as it may have rebound phenomena.
- Use TV only as a stress buster.
- Avoid contact with infections (e.g., chickenpox) and ensure age-appropriate vaccination.

Family support is vital. Parents should support and encourage the child to have realistic expectations and targets and facilitate undisturbed study time. They must avoid quarrels at any cost, should not make any unhealthy comparison, and resist the habit of constantly nagging the child on his/her study habits.

VIOLENCE AMONG YOUNG PEOPLE (10–24 YEARS) IS ON THE RISE

With the present-day philosophy of ends justifying means, it is only natural that the adolescents, the most vulnerable group of *Homo sapiens*, should resort to violence more and more to satisfy their real and perceived needs. At least some would claim that a child presenting with oppositional defiant disorder (ODD) and later on conduct disorder (CD) might be a candidate for adolescent violence. Children with CD have persistent dissocial, defiant, and aggressive behavior, and the three characteristic features of ODD are:

1. The range, frequency, and severity of disturbed behavior causing functional impairment.
2. Disregard of and contravention of normally accepted standards of behavior.
3. Failure to modify or desist from destructive behavior, despite persuasion or punishment.

MOOD DISORDERS ARE INCREASINGLY BEING RECOGNIZED

Mood disorders include depression (mood ↓↓), mania (mood ↑↑), or bipolar disorder with alternating high and low moods. Adolescent depression is often missed because parents may pass it off as normal adolescent mood changes. An adolescent may also try to mask depression with increased activity levels, so much so you may never find him/her with typical adult symptoms. To make any firm diagnosis of a psychiatric disorder, the age of onset of the symptom, duration, setting, and the impairment it has produced are all-important [Diagnostic and Statistical Manual of Mental Disorders, Fifth Edition (DSM-5) criteria].

It is often difficult to make the child and his/her parents understand "why to treat depression." We need to explain to them that there could be a primary neurotransmitter problem in the brain leading on to the mood changes and hence the need for drug therapy for about 6 months. Apart from this, they have biological symptoms of decreased or even increased appetite, less or disturbed sleep, and reduced interest in sexual matters. It may also be pointed out to the parents that on drug therapy, there is an increased chance for suicide, because the mood changes come only slowly, whereas the psychomotor retardation improves very rapidly, giving the person enough energy for suicidal act.

Cognitive behavioral therapy is indicated to overcome the cognitive error arising out of a defective thought process.

- *Cognitive error:* Overgeneralization, maximization of negative and minimization of positive attributes of the person
- *Thought process:* Irrational, illogical, and unrealistic.

Depression may be diagnosed in the school setting, using Beck's Depression Inventory (BDI). Studies by MKC Nair et al., have shown that among high school students, 3% have severe/extreme depression.

Interpretation of BDI is given in **Table 2**.

TABLE 2: Interpretation of Beck's Depression Inventory.

Score	*Interpretation*	*Suggested management*
0–10	Normal ups and downs	Nothing particularly
11–16	Mild mood disturbance	Group counseling in schools
17–20	Borderline depression	Individual counseling
21–30	Moderate depression	Individual counseling + medication as indicated
31–40	Severe depression	Medication + psychotherapy
>40	Extreme depression	Medication + psychotherapy

MENTAL HEALTH DISORDERS HAVE ONSET IN ADOLESCENCE

We have very few mental health specialists and too many mental health problems and hence there is a need for early detection programs in the community by health workers, family practitioners, pediatricians, and physicians. Fifty percent of mental disorders have onset before 14 years of age and 90% before 24 years of age. Common mental disorders are illustrated in **Table 3**.

DRUG THERAPY AND PSYCHOTHERAPY ARE A MUST FOR MENTAL HEALTH ILLNESSES

- *Severe/extreme depression:*
  - No improvement, atypical features
  - School refusal, substance abuse
  - Dysthymia—a long-standing depressed mood accompanied by loss of interest and lack of pleasure in usual enjoyable situations.

TABLE 3: Common mental disorders in children and adolescents.

Illness	*Identification and education*	*Action*
Intellectual disability	Delay in intellectual and adaptive functions	Referral
Autism	Deviation in social, communication, and imagination	Referral
ADHD	Inattention, restlessness; >6 months, two settings, onset before 12 years	Referral
Conduct disorder	Antisocial, defiant, aggressive	Referral
Anxiety disorder, obsessive compulsive disorder, post traumatic stress disorder	Obsessions, compulsions, trauma, recollections, avoidance, autonomic symptoms	Referral
Mood	Crying, suicidal, sleep, appetite less	Referral
Psychoses	Hallucination, delusion	Referral

(ADHD: attention-deficit/hyperactivity disorder)

Courtesy: Dr Paul Rusell, Professor and Head, Child and Adolescent Psychiatry Division, Christian Medical College, Vellore, Tamil Nadu.

- Conduct-disruptive and personality disorders
- High suicidal risk indicators present
- Psychosis with symptoms of:
    - *Hallucinations:* Seeing, hearing, smelling, or feeling—touch, unreal things/events
    - *Delusions:* Unshakable false belief
    - *Catatonic symptoms:* Fixed posture
    - Suicidal ideation or previous attempts.

Studies by Nair MKC et al., conducted in a *panchayat* among adolescent girls younger than 24 years of age showed that 85% of them justified suicide, provided there were adequate reasons like unwed pregnancy (42%), to prove innocence (28%), financial loss (17%), failed love affair (15%), and to counter parents (14%).

Mental Health Disorders: Psychopharmacology in a Nutshell

Medications for common mental disorders are outlined in **Table 4**.

TABLE 4: Psychopharmacology for children and adolescents.

Disorder	*Medication*	*Dose*	*Dosing*
ADHD	Atomoxetine	1.2–1.8 mg/kg	Once/twice daily
Anxiety disorder	Fluoxetine	10–40 mg	Once with breakfast
Depression	Fluoxetine	10–20 mg	Once with breakfast
Mania	Lithium + atypical antipsychotics	0.6–1 mmol/L	Once with dinner
Conduct disorder	Carbamazepine	8–12 mg/L	Once with dinner
Psychosis	Risperidone	2–4 mg/day	Once/thrice daily

(ADHD: attention-deficit/hyperactivity disorder)

Courtesy: Dr Paul Russell, Professor and Head, Child and Adolescent Psychiatry Division, Christian Medical College, Vellore, Tamil Nadu.

CONCLUSION

Adolescent mental health issues like autism, ADHD, learning disability may continue from childhood. These may be present for the first time in teenage as mental distress triggered by pubertal changes, parental conflicts, failed relationships, scholastic issues or as co-morbidity with mental disorders like depression, anxiety etc. Counseling is the mainstay of treatment in almost all adolescent behavioral and emotional issues. In a few cases with mental disorders depending on severity, medication may be needed.

SUGGESTED READING

1. Galagali P. Interviewing a teenager and anticipatory guidance using basic counselling skills. In: Patil G, Kanikar A, Luiz N, Chaterjee S (Eds). IAP-AHA Textbook of Adolescent Medicine. New Delhi: Jaypee Brothers Medical Publishers; 2024. pp. 40-4.
2. Galagali PM, Rao C, Dinakar C, Gupta P, Shah D, Chandrashekaraiah S, et al. Indian Academy of Pediatrics consensus guidelines for adolescent friendly health services. Indian Pediatr. 2022;59:477-84.
3. Kanikar AM, Bansal CP. Adolescent Counseling. In Adolescent Friendly Pediatric Practice. Ed: Pemde H, Ratna Kumari TL, Galagali PM, Velmurugan. Jaypee Brothers Medical Publishers; 2024. pp. 98-105.
4. Nair MKC, Kaur G. Self-counseling. In:Patil G, Kanikar A, Luiz N, Chaterjee S (Eds). IAP-AHA Textbook of Adolescent Medicine. New Delhi: Jaypee Brothers Medical Publishers; 2024. pp. 132-4.

2 SECTION

Fundamentals of Counseling

7 CHAPTER

Tips for History Taking and Mental State Examination

Vidhu Kumar, Preeti M Galagali

INTRODUCTION

History taking and mental status examination are pre requisites for making a diagnosis and formulating an individualised counseling and manangement plan for an adolescent presenting with behaviour issues. This chapter discusses the basics of psychosocial history taking and mental status examination.

BASIC ASPECTS OF INTERVIEW

- Use clear and culturally relevant language.
- Start with open questions and ask leading questions later on only.
- Listening is the key to a successful interview.
- Facilitative process should be adopted to get the best out of the person.
- Neutrality should be the hallmark; do not mix up with your personal values.
- A realistically reassuring approach only should be taken.
- Carefully halt digressions and then proceed with the relevant discussion.
- Sincerity and genuineness should be evident in your approach.

Do not try to establish cause for the adolescent's problems before examining him/her fully along the following lines

SCHEME OF HISTORY TAKING

Presenting Problems

The specific problem with which the child or adolescent has been brought with is the presenting problem.

History of Present Illness

- Full nature of the presenting symptom
- Inquire about associated symptoms likely to be related to the presenting problem (e.g., depressive symptoms in a child with school refusal)
- Leading questions on many of the common psychiatric problems can be probed—ask about features of psychosis, depression, learning disorder, etc.
- Ask about sleep and appetite.
- Any precipitating factors

History of Past Illness

- Past history of any similar problem
- Past history of any other behavioral problem
- Past history of medical illness or treatment

Family History of Mental Illness

- Ask about similar or other problems in the family.
- Ask about alcoholism and suicide in the family.
- Ask about any stressors or conflicts in the family.

Personal History

- Birth history
- Development of the child
- Peer relations
- Academics
- Conduct problems
- Sexuality
- Habits like alcohol use

Previous Temperament

- Interpersonal and social relations
- Prevailing emotions
- Energy and initiative
- Standards and morals

SCHEME OF EXAMINATION

Appearance and Behavior

- Dressing and grooming
- Eye contact
- Hyperactivity/hypoactivity
- Any strange behaviors

Examination of Thought

- Is the thought relevant?
- Examine for fears, ideas with undue emotional importance, negative thoughts, and strange and false ideas like delusions (unshakable false belief).

Examination of Perception

Examine for unusual perceptual phenomena like hallucinations (visual, auditory, olfactory, tactile, etc.).

Examination of Emotions

- What is the predominant emotional state the person is showing?
- Whether emotions are expressed less or more

Others, Like Memory, Intelligence

- Recent memory is more important, like "What happened yesterday?"
- Simple age-appropriate questions regarding arithmetic and general knowledge will give an idea about intelligence.

SCHEME OF DIAGNOSIS

- Due to medical disorder
- Due to substance abuse
- Psychotic disorder
- Mood disorder
- Anxiety disorder
- Somatoform and dissociative disorder

- Sexual and gender identity disorder
- Adjustment disorder
- Personality disorder

HEEADSSS PSYCHOSOCIAL HISTORY

HEEADSSS is a popular aid used globally by adolescent physicians to elicit a psychosocial history from an adolescent client. HEEADSSS is an acronym that stands for home, education/employment, eating, activities, drugs, sexuality, suicide, and safety. This tool is used to obtain history regarding these key issues. HEADSS was first developed by Henry Berman in 1972. In 1985, it was modified by Eric Cohen and its latest version was given by Goldenring and Rosen in 2004. They added an additional E for eating and S for safety. Another modified version HEADS/S F/FIRST is also in use that includes details regarding home, education, abuse, drugs, safety, sexuality, family, friends, image, recreation, spirituality, and threats.

Effective communication techniques should be used to elicit HEEADSSS. These include asking open-ended questions with a nonjudgmental and reflective listening attitude. This should be elicited in private. This will encourage bidirectional communication and make the adolescent feel at ease. The limits of confidentiality should also be explained to the client.

All the issues may not be explored at the first interview. Depending on the rapport formed with the client and availability of time, the interview can be split into three visits of 30 minutes each.

Home

Home is a vital part of an adolescent's life. For example, an adolescent who is being abused at home and is showing externalizing symptoms in the form of aggression and bullying will need help to keep himself/herself safe as well as require counseling and rehabilitation.

The questions will include details regarding family and family members, living conditions, privacy, and discipline issues. The strongest predictor of resilience is connectedness with a supportive trustworthy adult.

The questions that can be asked include the following:

- Who lives at home with you?
- How is your relationship with each family member?
- Do you share your problems with any family member?
- Do you have a separate room? Who gives you a bath?
- Do you sleep alone?
- Has there been a recent change in living arrangement?
- If I was invisible and you were having a disagreement with your parent, what would I hear? How would I see your parent disciplining you?

Education/Employment

Adolescents spend at least 6–8 hours in the school every day. Environment and connectedness at school have an impact on an adolescent's personality and resilience.

In India, scholastic issues regarding concentration, performance, and school behavior are one of the most common reasons for which an adolescent and his/her parents seek counseling. A recent decline in academic performance may suggest drug abuse, depression, bullying, sexual abuse, undiagnosed mild learning disability, and attention deficit. The questions should cover teacher and peer relations, study skills, recent and past academic performance, and goals for the future.

If the adolescent is working, details regarding his/her workplace and employers are elicited. According to the Child Labor Law, it is illegal to employ any child younger than 14 years.

The following questions can be asked:

- Are you studying/working?
- How is the situation at school/workplace?
- How has your performance been in school this year compared with the last? Are you satisfied with your performance?
- Are you a member of an educational club?
- How is your relationship with your teachers?
- How is your relationship with peers at school?
- Has anybody ever spoken to you in a way that you have not liked?

- Who helps you with schoolwork? Details regarding study habits and skills can be elicited.
- Where do you see yourself 5 years from now?

Eating

In India, there is a triple burden of malnutrition—undernutrition, obesity, and micronutrient deficiency. Most of the adolescent girls are anemic. Malnutrition has an adverse impact on the current and future health of adolescents; hence, it is essential to take a detailed nutritional history including intake of fruits, vegetables, and dairy products and calculate the calories and proteins consumed. Body image issues, indiscriminate snacking, and junk food intake can also be explored. A change in appetite may be a pointer toward depression or mania, diabetes, or brain tumor.

A few representative questions are as follows:

- How do you feel about your body?
- Recall your dietary intake on a typical day.
- How often do you eat out/drink colas?
- How do you stay healthy?
- What do you think about your diet?
- Do you ever feel that food controls you rather than vice versa?
- Has there been any change in your appetite lately?

Activities

An adolescent usually enjoys talking about his/her hobbies. Asking questions about the same enhances rapport building. It also gives an idea about the time spent in recreation, physical activity, television and computer viewing, sleep, peer-related activities, peer group, and extra academic strengths. Cocurricular and physical activities are essential for the physical and psychosocial well-being of an adolescent. Any recent loss in interest in activities may be a pointer toward unresolved emotional issues and depression. Peers have a great influence on the behavior of an adolescent. It is essential to know in detail about peers and peer-related activities like visit to pubs or drug usage. Adolescents may be exposed to inappropriate media messages regarding drugs, violence, body image issues, and sexuality.

Some of the questions that can be asked include the following:

- What do you do for fun?
- How much time do you spend in structured or unstructured outdoor/physical activity?
- For how long do you watch mobile and TV and use the computer? Do you have a TV and computer in your room? Do you own a mobile? What do you use media for? Which is your favorite media program/game? Are you a member of a social networking site? How do you feel after media use? Are you able to control your media use?
- What are your hobbies? Do you attend special hobby classes? Are you happy with your performance?
- Do you have friends you socialize with?
- Where do you and your peers hang around for fun?
- How is your relationship with friends?
- For how many hours do you sleep? Do you have any sleep-related problems?
- Have you lately lost interest in activities that you enjoyed previously?

Drugs

It is important to screen adolescents for drug abuse at every health visit. Drug use in adolescence can lead to lifelong addiction and permanent changes in the hippocampus that is associated with learning and memory. An adolescent may not answer in the affirmative to a direct questioning about drugs. Indirect query regarding drug use in friends may result in disclosure.

A few helpful questions to screen for drug use include the following:

- What is your attitude toward drug usage? How do you feel about this issue?
- Does any of your friends smoke, drink, or use drugs?
- Have you ever tried? If yes, which drug and how often?

Sexuality

Sexual health is often a sensitive issue for both adolescent and the healthcare provider. The sexual history should be taken in gender-neutral terms without making assumptions regarding the orientation of the adolescent.

The questions given next may be asked to elicit a history regarding sexual health, orientation, sexual abuse, and menstrual issues in girls. It is useful to begin the history taking with a "normalizing qualifier" statement like "I ask these questions from all young people. As your counselor, it is important for me to know about each and every aspect of your health".

- When did you attain menarche?
- What is the length of your menstrual cycle and for how long does the bleeding last? How many pads do you use in a cycle? Are you in a steady relationship? Have you been physically intimate with somebody? If yes, with whom?
- What do you do in intimate moments? How do you express your affection?
- Are you married?
- Do you use any contraceptive method?
- Have you ever been pregnant?
- Do you have any vaginal/penile discharge or itching?
- Do you have burning micturition?
- Has anybody touched you in a way that you did not like?

Suicide and Depression

Undiagnosed and untreated depression is a common cause of adolescent morbidity and mortality. Unlike adults, anhedonia may not be the cardinal feature. Depressed adolescents may present with irritability. It is also useful to ask insight questions to gain information regarding emotional needs and issues in a nonthreatening way. It is essential to inquire about suicide to enable early intervention by a referral to the psychiatrist.

The following questions could be asked:

- Have you ever felt hopeless, sad, and a failure in life?
- Has there been a recent change in your mood, behavior, sleep, appetite, or academic performance?
- On a scale of 10, rate your present mood. What would make you feel better?

- What do you do when you feel sad?
- Do you confide your problems in someone?
- Sometimes when young people are in unbearable pain or trouble, they wish that they could end it all. Have you ever wished the same? Have you ever tried to kill yourself?
- If someone gave you three wishes, what would they be?

Safety

Globally, injuries are the most common cause of adolescent mortality. Inquiries should be made regarding safety at home and school, vehicle usage, use of safety devices, and indulgence in violence. According to the Indian Motor Vehicle Act, young people above the age of 16 years can drive a 50cc vehicle with a learner's license and can get a regular license only after 18 years. Wearing of helmets is mandatory in most Indian states.

The following questions could be asked:
- Do you feel safe at home and school?
- Where do you play?
- Do you drive a vehicle? If yes, which one?
- Do you wear a helmet and seat belt while riding in a vehicle?
- Have you ever been in a physical fight? Have you ever got into trouble with the law?

Advantages of Eliciting a Psychosocial History

HEEADSSS is a useful tool for taking a comprehensive psychosocial history from an adolescent. The questions are structured in a manner that "less" sensitive issues like home, education, and activities are dealt with first and later "more" sensitive ones like sexuality and drugs are touched upon. This helps in developing rapport with the young person.

A few advantages are enumerated below:
- *Making a clinical diagnosis and prioritizing management issues and for follow-up:* Using HEEADSSS, the counselor can find pointers toward abuse, eating disorders, drug abuse, and depression in a quick and structured manner. If an adolescent

is getting abused, the first priority would be keeping him/her safe from further abuse. Thus, HEEADSSS clearly identifies the psychosocial areas of concern and thereby aids in intervention for appropriate case management. It also helps in follow-up counseling sessions.

- *Screening high-risk behavior and anticipatory guidance:* HEEADSSS screen provides an opportunity to the counselor in identifying high-risk behavior and providing anticipatory guidance regarding these important issues. For example, even though an adolescent does not use drugs, while talking about this issue, the counselor can inform the adolescent about the effect of drugs on the immature adolescent brain and methods to resist peer pressure.
- *Identifying strengths and strength-based counseling:* HEEADSSS can be used for positive youth development by identifying strengths in terms of developmental assets of mastery, independence, belonging, and generosity. For example, close family relationships indicate a sense of belonging, making healthy food choices shows independence, helping friends indicates generosity, and working with a tutor diligently is a pointer towards mastery. Strengths in one domain can be used to overcome weaknesses in another. Appreciating strengths helps in reinforcing them. This forms the basis of strength-based counseling. Identifying strengths can also be useful in motivational counseling.

CONCLUSION

A detailed psychosocial history facilitates the counseling process. It should be taken in private offering confidentiality. This helps to form a therapeutic alliance with the adolescents and their parents, identifies their concerns, strengths and vulnerabilities and helps in formulating goals for counseling. A mental status examination is essential to rule out and assess the severity of mental disorders and thereby the need for medication. History taking and mental status examination need to be repeated at follow up counseling sessions to assess recovery, duration and interval of sessions and termination.

SUGGESTED READING

1. Galagali P. Interviewing a teenager and anticipatory guidance using basic counselling skills. In: Patil G, Kanikar A, Luiz N, Chaterjee S (Eds). IAP-AHA Textbook of Adolescent Medicine. New Delhi: Jaypee Brothers Medical Publishers; 2024. pp. 40-4.
2. Galagali PM, Rao C, Dinakar C, Gupta P, Shah D, Chandrashekaraiah S, et al. Indian Academy of Pediatrics consensus guidelines for adolescent friendly health services. Indian Pediatr. 2022;59:477-84.
3. Klein M, Goldenring JM, Adelman W. (2014). HEEADSSS 3.0: the psychosocial interview for adolescents updated for a new century fuelled by media. Contemporary Pediatrics. [online] Available from https://www.contemporarypediatrics.com/view/heeadsss-30-psychosocial-interview-adolescents-updated-new-century-fueled-media [Last accessed September, 2024].

8 CHAPTER

Counseling Skills and Techniques

Sonny Jose

INTRODUCTION

In order to effectively counsel, the therapist requires a repertoire of skills and techniques. A skill is the learnt capacity or talent to carry out specific tasks in order to achieve predetermined results with the minimum outlay of time, energy, or both. A technique refers to a procedure used to accomplish a specific activity or task, and this chapter attempts to define the skill sets required for the counseling process.

Counseling is generally defined as a process in which a therapist (counselor) purposefully devotes her/his time and effort in order to assist a person in need (counselee) to consider her/his life situation to identify and act upon it, within the limitations of her/his environment. Characteristically, most definitions seem to suggest that counseling takes a systematic approach of the following:

- Assessing the problem/situation
- Ascertaining the root cause(s) of the problem (diagnosing)
- Identifying strategies and selecting a strategy (exploring)
- Implementing it
- Evaluating its outcomes.

RELATING–UNDERSTANDING–CHANGING FRAMEWORK IN COUNSELING

Counseling may be considered to be happening in three distinct phases—relating, understanding, and changing—referred to in the literature as the relating-understanding-changing (RUC) model/framework in counseling.

Relating Phase

Relating phase is the phase during which the therapist attempts to establish rapport, denotive of a professional working relationship.

Understanding Phase

The therapist attempts to understand the problem by partializing the problem, analyzing the cause–effect relationship, and understanding its implications to the client. Over and above, the therapist needs to communicate empathy for the client to feel listened to. It is also necessary in most cases to assist the client to handle her/his emotions.

Changing Phase

During this phase, the therapist needs to handhold the client into discerning what is desirable, decide on what to change and how to change, and commit to the same. Therefore, the most essential skills required to become an effective counselor may be related to these three stages **(Table 1)**.

Corresponding to the RUC model, it may be assumed that there are two skill subgroups: (1) Listening and attending, corresponding to the relating phase, and (2) counseling interventions, which correspond to the understanding and changing phases. Similarly, corresponding to various phases and skill subgroups, a set of skills is proposed. One should, however, note that many of the given skills are basic and not necessarily exhaustive. Second, the skills and the subgroups mentioned herewith need not be strictly considered to be watertight compartments.

TABLE 1: Three phases of counseling.

<table>
<tr><th>Phases</th><th>Skill subgroups</th><th>Skill sets</th></tr>
<tr><td>Relating</td><td>Attending and listening</td><td rowspan="3">• Attending and listening skills
• Responding skills
• Cathartic skills
• Decision-making skills
• Planning
• Closure skills</td></tr>
<tr><td>Understanding</td><td rowspan="2">Counseling interventions</td></tr>
<tr><td>Changing</td></tr>
</table>

ATTENDING AND LISTENING SKILLS

During the relating phase, the counselor is meeting the client, perhaps for the first time or during a subsequent follow-up. Here, it is important to make the client feel comfortable and predisposed to disclosure. To motivate the client to disclose, there are two prerequisites: First is the ambience of a nonthreatening atmosphere and the second is essentially the rapport indicative of the manner in which the client is handled by the therapist. The latter refers very much to the counselor's skills in attending as well as listening.

Considering the fact that the first impression is the best impression, the counselor has to make the first meeting (or even subsequent meetings) a positive experience. This is possible only if the counselor has established rapport with the client. The first set of skills, essentially required during this phase, is referred to as attending skills. Attending skills are necessary for the counselor to pay total attention to the client and at the same time becoming self-aware of herself/himself, in terms of the internal dialogue transacted within. Thus, the therapist is able to maintain a "therapeutic distance" that will save herself/himself the trouble of getting emotionally involved by transference or enmeshment. It also helps the counselor to engage the client, rather than appearing to be clinically distant.

Listening requires hearing by paying attention to every little communication made by the client. Listening in the context of counseling requires listening to the verbal expression by the client and its literal meaning. In addition to what is being said, the counselor has to be adept in reading between the lines, deciphering what "actually" is being said. It includes observation as well as listening skills. In short, listening refers to the conscious effort taken by the counselor to focus on the client (the other) by becoming aware of "what the other is saying" as well as "what the other is trying to communicate". True, the client speaks of many matters (linguistics) by way of words, phrases, metaphors, etc. Mehrabian was emphatic that hardly 7% of communication happens verbally. The major chunk of communication happens nonverbally by way of paralinguistics (intonation, volume, pitch, fluency, timing, mumbles, etc.) and the body language (gestures, facial expressions, posture, etc.). The paralinguistic accounts for as much as 38% of communication, while the body language accounts for 55%. For this, the therapist has to possess observation skills necessary to take note of nonverbal communications that essentially mirror the internal climate of the client and become the richest source of empathy. These reveal the client's energy level and feeling, and the degree of congruence between what is presented and her/his actual experience. At the same time, the counselor must essentially be able to communicate the empathy to the client. The above skills may be translated into action by way of certain techniques.

Techniques (Attending and Listening Skills)

Recording

It is advisable to record the transactions happening during a counseling session, combining narration and verbatim presentation, as required. Such a report would keep the counselor on target and be specific to the problem. A record would also allow continuity in the event of the client being transferred to or attended to by another counselor. It is important to note verbalization or specific problem presentations in the very language mentioned by the client. This would come in handy at the time of follow-up.

"Free-floating" Attention

In order to pay rapt attention to the client, the counselor needs to focus fully outside herself/himself, onto the client. For this to be possible, the counselor has to make note of every communication—verbal, paralinguistic, as well as nonverbal—attempt to experience each of them in terms of their different aspects (the intensity, frequency), and assess what each of them emotes. Thus, in many respects, the counselor gradually becomes absorbed by the client. However, the counselor must consciously become aware of his/her own personal thoughts and theorems and as far as possible evade going into these. Such fantasies keep him/her from understanding the other person, generally tend to distort the actual experience as presented by the client, and most often tell the counselor more about himself/herself than about the client.

Dos

- As far as possible, the counselor must keep himself/herself away from his/her internal domain consisting of his/her own thoughts, reactions, and feelings and should redirect attention onto the client.
- The counselor, while counseling, avoids internal constructs—"hunches"—or fantasy (ideas and beliefs) about the client and the problem presented. Such "internal dialogs" are understood to have no bearing on what is going on at the moment and are largely the counselor's attribution.

Minimal Use of Prompts

The therapist must use a varied repertoire of sounds and syllables to acknowledge that the client is being listened to. This includes a judicious use of prompts such as "mmm's", "uhuh's", "yes's" and even nonverbal communication in the form of nods.

SOLER

SOLER, as suggested by Egan, is an acronym that may be elaborated as follows:

- Sit squarely in relation to the client.
- Open position, to be maintained.
- Lean slightly toward the client.
- Eye contact, to be maintained reasonably.
- Relax.

Calibration

Calibration is a technique by which the counselor attempts to mirror and, to the maximum extent possible, empathize with the client. Here, the counselor as far as possible mirrors the client. This may be done by aligning the body posture, the tone and volume, and at a higher level even the breath rhythm. This may be possible by the following:

- Watching closely the client and posing as if a mirror image of the client
- Responding at the same pace, tone, and volume as the client

- Watching the shoulder movements of the client and pace of breathing in and out

RESPONDING SKILLS

Responding skills are also known as client-centered skills. The central assumption in a client-centered approach to counseling is the belief that individuals can change and want to change. In other words, it is assumed that the client is capable of making decisions about her/his own life and changing at her/his own pace. Furthermore, the counselor believes in the client's ability to find solutions; the therapeutic relationship process only enhances this ability. During the understanding phase, in addition to using attending and listening skills, the counselor is expected to assist the client in exploring the problem. This requires skills for probing and appropriately responding to the client.

While counseling, the counselor is expected to make minimal interventions, but at the same time elicit more frequent and appropriate responses from the client. Hence, questions need to be kept to the minimal while extracting the maximum. It would be good to remember that verbose does not help nor does it impress. Similarly, questions need to be used judiciously, only to explore, to elicit information, to clarify (did you say ... or....?), and to encourage the client to talk. In order to elicit maximum desirable response during a counseling session, the counselor is expected to ask a specific type of questions. The skill in this context is in asking the appropriate type of questions while avoiding the inappropriate ones.

Dos and Don'ts

Dos

Always ask the following:

- *Open questions:* It is important to include open-ended questions, also known as "open questions". Open questions open up the possibility of extracting elaboration with regard to any issue discussed instead of getting a "yes" or "no" answer. This helps in understanding the client and enhances the possibility of including the client's point of view. On the other hand, closed-ended questions limit the options to a "yes" or "no" answer, leading the counselor into a blind alley.

- *Example 1:* "Do you like Mallika?" (closed-ended question) versus "How do you feel about Mallika?" (open question)
- *Example 2:* "Do you do anything with your husband" (closed-ended question) versus "What kind of things do you do with your husband?" or "How do you generally spend time with your husband?" (open questions)

Don'ts

As far as possible, avoid asking the following:

- *Leading questions:* Leading questions are those type of questions that force the client to be (morally) wrong whichever way it is answered. Hence, such questions need to be suitably rephrased as demonstrated below:
  - *Example 1:* "Have you stopped beating your wife?"
    It is interesting to note that even with an answer in the affirmative "yes," it can still imply that the client had been beating his wife and now he has stopped. In any case, it implicates the client by answering the question. Instead, a better way would be to ask something such as "How do you deal with your wife now, when you get angry?"
  - *Example 2:* Imagine a client being asked "Do you feel guilty after masturbating?"
    His answer, whether it be a "yes" or "no", still does not reveal whether indeed the client is engaging in such an act. A "no" might mean that the client does not feel guilty or simply the fact that the client is not even doing it. Similarly, a "yes" might only reflect his morality, even if he was not engaging in such an act. Hence, a softer option would be to ask, "How do you feel after masturbating?"
- *Value-laden questions:* These questions not only speculate the counselor's value system but also further pose a moral question and guarantee that the client is indisposed in answering them.
  - *Example 1:* Imagine the counselor is met by a young lady client who confesses that she had been jilted by her

lover. It would be natural for the counselors to explore the relationship. By sheer logic, the counselor would not hesitate asking, "What did he do to hurt you?", "Can you tell me about your life with him?", "I'm sorry ... did he treat you so badly?", etc. But imagine in actuality she was a lesbian; what would be her predicament other than withdrawing? Obviously, here the counselor has thrust his value system onto the client and has measured the client to his/her standards.

  - *Example 2:* To a question such as "Are you guilty of your homosexuality?", the natural and logical answer is a "yes", since answering in the negative is considered not to be socially desirable. Instead, the counselor may present the issue in such a way that the client thinks, reflects, and answers. Hence, the question may be "What do you feel about your sexual orientation?" or "What sort of dilemmas do you encounter being a gay?" and go on to explore the details.

- *Either-or questions:* Such questions instead of presenting the client the options often expose the concerns (or even the dilemmas) of the counselor. Asking either-or questions actually limit the options of the client to the counselor's preference. A typical either-or question would sound as follows:
  - *Example 1:* "Would you like to talk about your job or marriage today?" Instead, the options are broadened if the counselor was to ask the client, "What issue would you like to discuss today?" Or in another instance, suppose the client is asked, "Have you and Jimmy decided to get married or have an abortion?" Such a question not only reveals the counselor's priorities but also undermines the morale of the client, if ever he/she had other more important matters to be considered for discussion. A better question would be, "What alternatives have you and Jimmy talked about?"
- *Suggestive questions:* These questions hint at a "desired" answer and convey conditions. The latter violates the principle of self-determination (in social work) of the client as well as goes against the counseling principles. Typical examples are given as follows:
  - *Example 1:* "Don't you think it is high time you gave up drinking and shaped up?"

Such a question suggests the ideals as perceived by the counselor. These need not be the client's priorities and hence would turn him/her against the counselor. Instead, it may be made more exploratory and less implicating. The better option would be to ask, "Do you think you have a drinking problem?" or "What would you like to do about your drinking binge?"

- *"Why?" questions:* "Why?" questions almost remind the client of being in the dock. Such questions would turn the counseling session into an interrogation. Hence, they may at best be avoided.
- *Confronting questions:* Confrontation or direct questioning might sour up the relationship, if not used gently and appropriately. Hence, confrontation need only be used after the therapeutic relationship deepens and the client is comfortable with the counselor as well as his/her intentions.
- *Bombarding (or double-barreled questions):* At times, the counselor, not being clear about what to ask or for reasons of overeagerness, asks the client more than one question. Such double-edged questions confuse the client, especially if he/she has to answer one in the affirmative and the other in the negative. A classic example would be to ask:
  - *Example 1:* "How are you feeling today and did you get a chance to discuss with your wife what we had talked about last week?"
  - *Example 2:* "What were your parents' reactions when you talked about being pregnant? Did they suggest abortion? How do you feel about having an abortion?"

    Instead, break it down, and ask them one by one.

Techniques (Responding Skills)

Some good techniques are given in the following text in order to facilitate better responses from the client as well as aid understanding (as in the RUC model).

Funneling

Funneling is the systematic and gradual process of moving from a general area to something very specific. By funneling, the counselor assists the client to explore the areas he/she wants to explore. In the below-given verbatim, one may note how the counselor skillfully moves from a general feeling of upset experienced by the client to the specific problem that concerns his/her son Kamal:

Counselor: "You seem upset at the moment ... what is happening?"

Client: "Emmm ... its home ... things aren't working out".

Counselor: "What is happening at home?"

Client: "I'm falling out with Janu and the children".

Counselor: "What does Janu feel about what is happening?"

Client: "She's angry ... with me of all people".

Counselor: "About something in particular?"

Client: "Yes ... about the way I deal with my son, Kamal".

Counselor: "What is the problem with Kamal?"

Reflection

Reflection is the process of "echoing" back onto the client what the counselor gathers from the conversation. It is important to calibrate in terms of tone and voice of the client's. This technique helps to maintain the locus of control of the relationship on the client.

Client: "We lived in Kerala for a few years ... initially things were exciting ... then suddenly everything collapsed".

Counselor: "What collapsed?"

Client: "Well ... we never really settled ... my wife missed her parents and home town ... I too did ... But we never really talked about it."

Counselor: "Neither of you admitted that you missed your friends ... and you never talked about it?"

Client: "I guess we really did not want to admit it ... if I admitted, I would be letting the other person down ... I guess we wanted to protect each other".

Selective reflection: Often, clients make subtle, throw-away remarks about something they are emotionally charged about. Selective reflection refers to the manner of putting back to the client something they emphasized in between or seems to be emotionally charged about. This requires the keen attention and involvement of the counselor. However, the counselor has to learn to keep the conversation seamless and contextual. The following is a verbatim from a conversation with an IT couple:

Client: "We married very young ... money came in ... we bought this huge flat ... but she never seemed to like it ... she hated it ... I thought it important to start somewhere."

Counselor: "Your wife hated the flat?" (selective reflection)

Empathy Building

Sometimes, the client hesitates to come to the point and tends to beat around the bush. With such clients, the counselor intuitively understands what the client is experiencing and puts it back to the client in a direct manner. In doing so, it is more important to understand what is implied rather than explicit.

Client: "People at work are just the same ... they are uptight and tied with their own things ... life, friends and family ..."

Counselor: "You sound angry with them" (intuition).

Client: "I suppose so ... they don't bother to ask how I am getting on."

Counselor: "It sounds that you are saying that they haven't had time for you for long" (intuition).

Client: "They haven't ... my family hasn't bothered much ... they look as if they are ... but they are not."

Clarifying (Paraphrasing)

In this technique, the counselor checks for understanding by asking the client whether he/she has been understood correctly. Clarification is done by summarizing occasionally in order to clarify what is being said.

Client: "I feel all over the place ... things aren't just right ... money is a problem and work ...."

Counselor: "Let me just clarify .... You mean to say, you have been planning to quit work."

CATHARTIC SKILLS (SKILLS TO HELP WITH FEELINGS)

In counseling, a considerable amount of time is spent on working with "feelings" or emotional content. To complicate matters, emotions are culture specific, free expression often frowned upon, leading to "bottling up." Emotions blocked within tend to cause physical discomfort as they become trapped in muscular clusters. This in the long-term causes breathing, musculature, and postural problems, as well as psychosomatic illnesses. Another dimension to emotion is the ambivalence. Individuals are unable to differentiate and label the mixed feelings that they encounter. Furthermore, intense and ambivalent emotions cloud the mind and render the individual incapable of arriving at rational decisions. Bottling up of emotions manifests as follows:

- Faulty self-image due to repression, unexpressed grief
- Setting unrealistic targets
- Doing unrealistic things (as in a fit of anger), forcing failure
- Clouding of perception, e.g., women are infidel, all people cheat you
- Last straw syndrome—"displacement" and/or purging out emotions on others after continuous repression

Techniques (Cathartic Skills)

Acknowledging

Emotions being cultural specific, often the client requires some kind of an assurance from the part of the counselor to express them. Even while crying, clients attempt to hold back their tears in embarrassment of being seen crying. A good therapist must realize the value of expression and must acknowledge the client and give permission to cry. The counselor might have to be as explicit as stating, "It's ok with me, for you to cry."

Reliving

Reliving is a powerful tool of revisiting the past experience. While doing this technique, the counselor assumes the role of a therapist by taking the client down the memory lane to explore the event. Specific memory cues such as time, place, person(s), and event, as well as sensory cues of visual, auditory, tactile, olfactory, and kinesthetic stimuli, have to be included in order to relive the previous experience.

Alter Ego

Here, the client (ego) is seated with a person, opposite to each other. First, the client is encouraged to freely express what he/she has to the person. Next, the client and the person exchange seats and the fellow (alter ego) mimics the client's expression back onto the client. This gives the client an opportunity to take a look at his/her own perspective and understand the implications of the same. A discussion and feedback between the client (ego) and the person (alter ego) that ensues allows the client to emerge with a fresh perspective and a better adaptive behavior.

Empty Chair

During the empty chair exercise, the client is made to imagine striking a conversation with the person/situation in which they have been involved. Special attention is paid to addressing the feeling.

Counselor: "How do you feel like?"

Client: "I feel like a bobbin case badly mixed up ..."

Counselor: "What does the bobbin case say to you?"

Client: "It says ... I want to keep you from making crucial decisions as long as possible."

Counselor: "What does it imply?"

Client: "Guess ... I want to delay meeting the opponent in the court ... don't know whether I will be able to hold off my anger ..."

Exaggeration

In this technique, the therapist helps in locating a physical experience within and invites the client to explore the same in order to locate an event in the remote memory.

Counselor: "What are you feeling at this moment …?"

Client: "I feel an emptiness …"

Counselor: "Where do you feel that emptiness?"

Client: "Here …" (indicating the pit of the stomach)

Counselor: "Can you increase the feeling …?"

Client: "Yes, … it's spreading up my chest …"

Counselor: "Have you felt this way before?"

Client: "Yes … quite some time back when I went to the boarding."

Counselor: "What happened then?"

Client: "I felt empty … when separated from my sister …"

Mobilization of Body Energy

Bioenergetics acknowledges the fact that psychosomatic illnesses, as well as the body musculature, correspond to the emotions bottled (e.g., a hunch, curl up). Using this technique, the counselor lets the client experience the bottled-up emotion and later release the tension by stretching and breathing out.

Exploring Fantasy

Through this exercise, the counselor encourages the client to work the imagination to the limits. Considering the tendency among individuals to avoid a negative scenario, the client is asked to imagine and experience the "worst-case scenario." This would help the client to understand perhaps that it was not as bad as he/she imagined, e.g., if afraid of going on stage or to an interview, letting them imagine and experience the worst, e.g., seeing them trembling, stammering, dropping the notes, or even falling unconscious.

Rehearsal/Role Playing

Here, the client is coached by the counselor to take roles that he/she is uncomfortable with. Such a rehearsal provides invaluable exercise, especially when preparing a person to face a situation with renewed confidence, e.g., coaching a timid individual for asserting himself before the boss, providing a mock interview to help the candidate face the interview with improved body language, or teaching a teenager on how to resist sexual advances by the peers.

DECISION-MAKING SKILLS

Now that the client has experienced catharsis by expressing his/her feelings, the client becomes more rational. At this stage, he/she is more predisposed to decision-making. The counselor assists the client in exploring plausible strategies in order to resolve the problem. Having considered the options, the client is made to commit to one particular strategy that is considered the most desirable. At the other extreme, for a client with little options or experiencing an avoidance—avoidance dilemma (in which both options are equally unacceptable), the client is made to select the least damaging option (based on the "doctrine of lesser evil").

Techniques (Decision-making Skills)

Force-field Rating

The client is made to weigh the pros and cons of each decision. Each of these is written down and assigned a specific value, let us say, on a 10-point scale. The grand total (rating) of the pros and cons is considered and based on the scores a rational decision is made; for example, imagine you were approached by a friend who is in a dilemma about marriage. A software engineer in her own merit, she has got two marriage proposals at hand. Both appear to be equally attractive. But she can marry only one! In force-field rating, she is asked to consider each of the candidates, based on their merits and demerits, and rate them. We need to consider the difference between the merits and demerits (merits "minus" demerits).

TABLE 2: Example of force-field rating.

Infosysian				*Titan*			
Merit		***Demerit***		***Merit***		***Demerit***	
• Handsome • Teetotaler	• 8.5 • 9	• Tours	7	• MS from the United States • Handsome • Sociable	• 10 • 6 • 5	• Job-hopper • Too fastidious • Smoker	• 4 • 8 • 5
Net	17.5		7		21		17
Total	10.5						

In the example in **Table 2**, the Infosysian wins by a clear margin. You may use weightages for the parameters if the scores are inching close and of course if your mathematics is good!

Modeling

You may have clients whom you can make consider options. There are, however, clients who are unable to make decisions. For such clients, the counselor may consider the following options in the sequence suggested, i.e., if one does not work, go onto the next higher order:

- Ask the client to recall what he/she tried when the problem (or a similar problem) occurred last. Explore the options he/she made and attempt to explore additional ones, considering the fact that he/she is more logical and better equipped after catharsis. Assist him/her in fine-tuning a more effective strategy.
- Ask him/her to imagine that the same problem is happening to someone he/she respects and considers very mature. Ask what this "respectable" person would do if a similar problem occurred. Ask him/her to consider that option.
- If the client is thoroughly "incapable", the counselor may share what his/her other clients did in similar situations and ask him/her whether any of the options pro-offered would work, given his/her circumstances and limitations.
- The counselor should never advise and ask the client to follow her/his solution to the problem. As a last option, the counselor

may recommend certain other options (never one!) which he/she thinks might be feasible. Let the client explore these and decide.

PLANNING SKILLS

Planning implies laying a blueprint for action. For this to happen effectively, one may have to plan *SMART* (borrowed from project management and planning). The acronym expands to *s*pecific, *m*easurable, *a*chievable, *r*ealistic, and *t*ime bound.

Techniques (Planning Skills)

Planning SMART

In order to plan SMART, ask the client what he/she would want to achieve. In order to achieve what is planned, ascertain the following:

- Objectives to be achieved
- What are the possible tasks (actions) or even subtasks to be undertaken; weed out those unachievable, unrealistic, and the impossible!
- Decide on a time frame.
- Assign resources—material, money, and social support.
- Agree on checkpoints at various timings in order to cross-check whether the tasks have been accomplished and the objective realized.

Contracting

In the case of clients in a crisis or even suicide prone, it is good to keep a tab on. In the case of a client with suicidal behavior, it would be reassuring if the counselor does safety planning along with the client detailing healthy coping strategies, safety net of people with contact numbers and reasons for living. Other pacts include an agreement to call up the counselor and report on the developments after the last session. Remember that it is very important to agree upon a time; for example, in the case of a client with suicide proneness, the client is asked to call up and report at a specific time. A time sequence works like an alarm and elicits a time-tabled response which may be vital in sustaining a person in crisis. Second, given a number, the brain is tuned to accomplishing or meeting the suggested deadlines. Finally, the client is reassured of the counselor's concern.

CLOSURE SKILLS

Any process must be logically concluded. Just as it is presumed that the first impression is the best impression, the last impression makes a lasting impression. The focus in this stage is to put down everything with utmost clarity, preferably in black and white. Among the few things to be undertaken at closure, evaluation and planning are important and so are follow-up and termination.

Gentle Confrontation

As in the beginning, it is very important to evaluate the session. Typically, most individuals coming to a counselor are quite unlikely to acknowledge that they have changed. A client who is generally pessimistic or even reluctant to acknowledge change needs to be confronted. In confronting, as a principle, there should be conclusive evidence. This evidence can be had from the case sheet prepared during the initial interview. The best way of confronting would be to painstakingly go through each of the verbalizations in the same manner (colloquial) mentioned by the client. Thus, finally a person who initially remarks that there is "no change at all" would acknowledge reasonable change.

Scheduling

It is important to schedule a treatment regimen. Most professionals—medical as well as psychologist—lag in scheduling. The most practical sequence may be as given in **Table 3**.

TABLE 3: The most practical sequence.

First follow-up session	1 week after the first cluster of sessions
Second follow-up session	2 weeks (14 days) after first follow-up
Third follow-up session	3 weeks (21 days) after second follow-up
Fourth follow-up session	4 weeks (30 days) after third follow-up
Fifth follow-up session	6 weeks (45 days) after fourth follow-up

It is interesting to note that women generally abide by the (strict) regimen suggested by the counselor. However, men are less inclined to do so. Hence, it would be important to put down in writing the date for the next follow-up meeting.

CONCLUSION

Counseling, in order to be transacted effectively, requires the counselor to be adept on various fronts. The adeptness comes from being skilled and being able to translate the skills in practice using techniques. Hence, the counselor would have to consciously develop and acquire matching skills ranging from attending, listening, responding, cathartic, and decision-making to planning and finally closure. Similarly, he/she needs to put into practice appropriate techniques. These are essential in order to achieve predetermined results with the minimum outlay of time and energy. Considering the fact that the clients and their circumstances and problems are unique, the counselor needs to mix and match the skills and techniques depending on each case presented. However, one needs to understand that these skills and techniques cited are not exhaustive and present the opportunity for practitioners to adapt the same from diverse fields.

SUGGESTED READING

1. Burks H, Stefflre B (Eds). Theories of Counseling. New York: McGraw-Hill Education; 1979.
2. Burnard P. Counseling Skills for Health Professionals, 2nd edition. London: Chapman and Hall; 1994.
3. Carkhuff R. The Art of Helping, 4th edition. Massachusetts: Amhearst; 1983.
4. Egan G. The Skilled Helper. California: Brooks and Cole Publishing Company; 1994.
5. Epting TR. Personal Construct Counselling and Psychotherapy. Chichester: Wiley; 1984.
6. Feltham C, Dryden W. Dictionary of Counseling. London: Whurr; 1993.
7. Lowen A, Lowen L. The Way to Vibrant Health: A Manual of Bioenergetic Exercises. New York: Harper and Row; 1977.
8. Murgatroyd S. Counseling and Helping. London: British Psychological Society; 1986.

9. Nelson-Jones R. Introduction to Counseling Skills, 2nd edition. London: Sage; 2005.
10. Skill. [online] Available from http://en.wikipedia.org/wiki/Skills [Last accessed September, 2024].
11. Technique. [online] Available from http://en.wikipedia.org/wiki/Techniques [Last accessed September, 2024].

9 CHAPTER

Effective Counseling Model

Rev TJ Thomas

INTRODUCTION

The conceptual model presents three aspects of effective counseling: (1) Phases of the process, (2) goals of both counselor and counselee in each phase, and (3) skills required by the counselor for the achievement of the goals in each phase. The model is developmental and presents a prehelping phase and three stages of the process of counseling, that have been detailed in chapter 8.

PREHELPING PHASE—ATTENDING

The prehelping phase (attending/expressing) refers primarily to the counselor. The counselee may not consciously initiate the process by asking for help. In performance assessment sessions, the educator must be attentive to personally significant statements such as "I don't know what is going on"; "it just happens"; "why would he say that?"; etc. On being aware of such expressions, the counselor can then focus attention on the person trying to reveal a problem.

Counselor's Goal in Attending

The counselor's goal in attending is to attend to the counselee, both psychologically and physically, and to focus awareness on the verbal and nonverbal expressions of the counselee.

Counselor's Skill in Attending

A counselor's skill in attending is to listen attentively. The counselor, by his/her posture, lets the counselee know that he/she is available to him/her, that he/she is "with him/her" now. This is physical attending. The counselor listens attentively to both the verbal and the nonverbal messages of the counselee to whom he/she is available. Nonverbally, he/she listens to the messages that are carried in the counselee's tone of voice, silences, pauses, gestures, facial expressions, and posture. This is psychological attending. In summary, the counselor now focuses his/her attention on the following questions: What is this person communicating about himself/herself? About his/her feelings? About his/her thinking? And about his/her behavior?

PREHELPING PHASE—EXPRESSING

- *Stage I:* Responding/self-exploration
- *Stage II:* Integrative understanding/dynamic self-understanding
- *Stage III:* Facilitation action/acting

Stage I: Responding/Self-exploration

While attending to a student, or another person, the counselor becomes aware that the counselee has expressed something personally significant. Then he/she responds in a way that helps the counselee explore his/her behavior (his/her feelings, his/her attitudes, what he/she does, what he/she fails to do, what is constructive in his/her life, what is destructive, etc.).

Counselor's Goal in Responding

To respond to the counselee—what all counselor has to say (with empathy, genuineness, and respect) to establish rapport (a trusting collaborative working relationship) in order to facilitate the counselee's self-exploration.

The skills given in the following text are required by the counselor in order to facilitate the counselee's self-exploration.

Counselor's Skills in Responding

- *Empathic understanding:* The counselor responds to the counselee in a way that shows he/she has listened and that he/she understands what the counselee is saying about himself/herself and what he/she is feeling. In some sense, he/she tries to see the counselee's world from the counselee's frame of reference.

It is not enough to understand; the counselor communicates responsively his/her empathic understanding.

- *Respect:* The way in which the counselor responds should show that he/she respects the counselee. He/she communicates the very deepest respect for the counselee's worth as a person and for the counselee's potentials to be developed.
- *Genuineness:* The counselor is open and spontaneous in his/her responding. He/she is just another human being to the counselee sitting before him/her and is transparent in his/her concern.
- *Concreteness:* When the counselee rambles or speaks in generalities, the counselor grounds the helping process in concrete feelings and concrete behavior. The counselor communicates in ways showing how to focus on specifics.

The skills of stage I are crucial. If the counselor does not have them, he/she simply cannot help, because the skills of stages II and III are built on them. The ways in which empathic understanding, respect, and genuineness are expressed may change somewhat as the counselor moves on into the helping process, but the need for these skills continues throughout the process.

Counselee's Goal in Self-exploration

The goal is to explore his/her experience, behavior, and feelings relevant to the problems in his/her life; to explore the ways in which he/she is now living ineffectively.

Utilizing the responses of the counselor, the counselee expands his/her awareness of himself/herself. In the process, he/she clarifies issues, begins to recognize patterns in behavior, and becomes conscious of feelings in relation to failures, needs, and goals. While not an end in itself, self-exploration is necessary to reach self-understanding, which is the foundation for change reflected in action.

Stage II: Integrative Understanding/Dynamic Self-understanding

As the person receiving help explores the various problem areas in his/her life, he/she produces a great deal of data that are useful to the degree that they can be pieced together to reveal behavior patterns in his/her life. He/she begins to understand himself/herself in ways that were not apparent before. He/she begins to own responsibility for his/her thoughts, feelings, and actions. He/she experiences insight.

Counselor's Goal in Integrative Understanding

The goal is to understand and fit together the data produced by the counselee; to see and help the counselee identify behavioral themes; to help the counselee see the "large picture" (interactive understanding).

Counselor's Skills in Integrative Understanding

All the skills of stage I, plus the following:

- *Facilitative self-disclosure:* The counselor shares his/her own experience to the extent that it will actually help the counselee understand himself/herself. The counselor is free and spontaneous in volunteering personal information about himself/herself, provided this communication is constructive in facilitating the client to a deeper self-understanding (however, remember that the general rule is not to disclose the counselor's personal information).
- *Immediacy of relationship:* The counselor is willing to explore his/her own relationship with the counselee ("you–me" talk) to explore the here and now of counselor–counselee interactions, to the degree that it helps the counselee get a better understanding of himself/herself, of this interpersonal style, and of how he/she is utilizing the helping process.
- *Confrontation:* The counselor speaks specifically about discrepancies, distortions, and inconsistencies in the counselee's life (remember, keep confrontation to the minimum).

Counselee's Goal in Integrative Understanding

The goal is dynamic self-understanding, to develop understanding that sees the need for change, for action, learning the skill of putting together the larger picture for himself/herself; identifying resources, especially unused resources.

Ideally, as stage II progresses, the counselee sees more and more clearly the necessity for action on his/her part. He/she might be fearful of change and may doubt whether he/she has the resources necessary for change. These fears and doubts must be dealt with, if he/she is to act. Sometimes he/she needs to be supported to act first, in order to learn that his/her fears and doubts are baseless. The dynamic self-understanding sought in stage II may be defined as insight that leads to action programs.

Stage III: Facilitation Action/Acting

Effective counseling leads ultimately to changes in behavior. The procrastinator meets any deadlines comfortably; persons in conflict work through to resolution; passive persons take initiative; etc. In this final stage, the counselor and counselee work together in such a way that the counselee experiences satisfaction in living effectively.

Counselor's Goal in Facilitating Action

The goal is to collaborate with the counselee in working out specific action programs, so as to stimulate the counselee to act on his/her new understanding of himself/herself; to explore with the counselee a wide variety of alternatives for engaging in constructive behavioral change; and also to give support and direction to action programs.

Counselor's Skills in Facilitating Action

- All the skills of stage I, plus all the skills of stage II
- Developing action programs, utilizing problem-clarifying and problem-solving approaches, decision-making processes, program-planning models, and training in interpersonal skills.

Counselee's Goal in Facilitating Action

This may mean stopping some self-endangering activity, like absenteeism. This may also mean starting on some program for growth, i.e., a physical fitness program. This may mean developing new attitudes, such as a sense of self-worth through the conscious monitoring of accomplishments. Someone may decide to "talk things over with the boss". If so, the learning of communication skills may be a prerequisite program. The results of effective counseling are revealed in action or changes in behavior.

In most cases, the counselor and the counselee collaborate in both the elaboration of action plan and the working through of problems that may arise as the programs are pursued. If action programs require prior skills training, the counselor may train the counselee himself/herself or refer him/her to someone else. If a referral is made, it is important that the counselor maintain contact with the counselee and support him/her through the skills training program.

POSTCOUNSELING PHASE (CELEBRATION)

In this phase, satisfaction and fulfilment is experienced by the counselor and the counselee. As effective counseling results in effective living by the counselee, this spontaneously leads to some celebration. Awkward effort at expressing appreciation on the part of the counselee should be best met with a cup of tea or coffee. It is also transition time toward discontinuing the "counseling" relationship, as well as the other role as an educator.

CONCLUSION

A counselor needs to imbibe the skills of both attending and expressing to form a therapeutic alliance with the adolescent. Next the counselor leads the adolescent on the path of self awareness, integration and understanding of the problem and finally towards behavior change that leads to resolution of mental distress and termination of the counseling process. These form important components of an effective counseling process.

SUGGESTED READING

1. Galagali P. Interviewing a teenager and anticipatory guidance using basic counselling skills. In IAP- AHA Textbook of Adolescent Medicine. Jaypee Brothers Medical Publishers; 2024. pp. 40-44.

2. Galagali P. Child abuse: Recognition, Response and Counseling. In Safe Childhood–Right of every Child. Ed: Ashok Kumar, Rajeev Seth, Aby Dany Verghese. Published by Indian Child Abuse, Neglect and Child Labour Group of IAP. 2024; pp. 59-73.
3. Kanikar AM, Bansal CP. Adolescent Counselling. In Adolescent Friendly Pediatric Practice. Ed: Pemde H, Ratna Kumari TL, Galagali PM, Velmurugan. Jaypee Brothers Medical Publishers. 2024; pp. 98-105.

10 CHAPTER

Legal and Ethical Issues

Raghavendra Kumar K

INTRODUCTION

Since the prevalent laws can vary between countries, this chapter will help the counselors to be informed about a broader approach and general principles pertaining to medicolegal/ethical issues in India only. However, deciding on an approach to deal with specific minor details in the face of medicolegal/ethical matters, which one might encounter in due course of one's practice is beyond the scope of this chapter. Counselors are advised to consult a qualified medicolegal consultant in such a situation.

The first part of the chapter discusses certain key concepts/definitions which are vital for any person in the field of mental health or allied disciplines, such as "best interest of the child"; legality, ethicality, privacy, confidentiality, privilege; "need to know"; and "right to know".

The second part deals with the challenges a counselor can face in dealing with these issues and with the approach to those challenges.

KEY DEFINITIONS/CONCEPTS

- *Best interest of the child:* This principle is embodied in Article 3(1) of the United Nations Convention on the Rights of the Child (UNCRC), which states that "in all actions concerning children, whether undertaken by public or private social welfare institutions, a court of law, administrative authorities, or legislative bodies, the best interests of the child shall be a primary consideration".
- *Legality:* Here, the law has clearly enunciated codes/rules on a matter, and there are clear/well-defined consequences for not following these codes/rules.

- *Ethicality:* It is the moral code of conduct guiding a person's behavior. A simple rule of thumb for an ethical behavior is for us to behave in the way we would expect others to behave with us in a certain situation.
- *Privacy:* It is the inalienable *legal and ethical* right held by any individual to keep his or her matters related to personal and/or interpersonal issues secret. In the context of counselors dealing with children and adolescents, the legal rights of children under 18 years of age are vested in their parents/guardians/caregivers. This is one of the major sources of dilemmas arising while counseling children and adolescents. For instance, a child confiding in the counselor reveals having experimented with smoking. How would one as a counselor navigate this dilemma without antagonizing any of the stakeholders?
- *Confidentiality:* It is the unwavering *moral/ethical* commitment by the counselors/counselors to respect the privacy of a person who confides in them. In the above-mentioned instance of the child confiding in a counselor, revealing the experimentation with cigarettes to the parent/teacher can be detrimental to the therapeutic relation.
- *Privilege:* This is the legal right held by clients/their legal guardians for protecting them from their private information being divulged in judicial proceedings. This concept can vary based on the prevailing legal provisions of the countries/states and unfortunately in India there are no prevalent laws which talk about "privilege". On the contrary, there are laws which are binding on the counselor/counselor which ask for *mandatory reporting* of information which has come to the cognizance of the counselor. In the above-mentioned example, if the child were to confide about being sexually abused, instead of having experimented with cigarettes, it becomes a legal obligation of the person who becomes cognizant of the information to reveal it to concerned authorities. Failure to do so is punishable under Section 21 of the Protection of Children from Sexual Offences Act.

  Need to know: This concept is where information is revealed to a concerned person/organization in relevant parts. In the previously cited example, if the child is experimenting with cigarettes at school, along with peers (and especially when it is being made available at/around the school), and if the school counselor becomes cognizant of the information, it is ethically binding on the counselor to report the principal in the larger interest of several children at risk. In addition, as an employee of the school, the school may insist on knowing certain information. However, there is no legal binding in any manner. Here, the counselor can choose to reveal information in a manner which does not jeopardize the therapeutic relation. Even parents are ethically entitled to know in these circumstances.

- *Right to know:* This concept has been defined as the entitlement to be appraised of certain information by the concerned authorities like courts or police, as a part of their investigative process. This is different from *mandatory reporting*; the statutory bodies are vested with the rights to demand for the information obtained by the counselor in the process of therapeutic interactions, in the form of either summons or session notes.

The following section deals with the challenges a counselor can face in his or her daily practice and means to navigate those challenges.

BOUNDARIES

Boundaries with Other Professionals

Although it may seem simple to work as a team, it can get challenging if a team member wades into another person's area of expertise. Especially, when it comes to cases involving crimes against children, multidisciplinary team members, law, police, prosecutors, counselors, and child protective service providers frequently experience intense and challenging emotions. To avoid going too far and creating further problems, all team members need to uphold professional boundaries. It is important to keep in mind that each team member feels a variety of emotions, many of which are connected to certain tasks and ideas.

In addition, a counselor's level of emotional involvement is higher due to their ongoing concern for the child or adolescent client and/or the impact they have on the family.

Dos

- Do show politeness.
- Please state the facts.
- Please direct any inquiries about investigations to the prosecutor or law enforcement/other concerned authorities.
- Recognize that detectives work long hours and that every case needs specifics.
- Recognize that a thorough study requires time.

Don'ts

- Don't venture into legal matters on your own.
- Don't forecast or guarantee a particular result/outcome.
- Never presume to know what another professional is doing or when they will finish.
- Don't ask the parents or guardians for private information or specifics.

The likelihood of a successful conclusion is significantly raised when the team members develop strong, functional connections in which they recognize and complement each other's unique roles. It is crucial that team members cooperate with one another rather than against one another. For the investigation and prosecution process to proceed well, the interdisciplinary team's members must communicate effectively with one another. It should always be kept in mind that each of these professionals shares as his or her primary responsibility for serving children, adolescents, and their families, even though the functions of law enforcement, prosecutors, counselors, and others are somewhat different in this regard.

What needs to be kept in mind is that the "best interest of the child" is central in all the endeavors of all the professionals working with children.

Boundaries with Adolescents

Subtle instances that may represent a risk for boundary conflicts may occur during any counseling process. Adolescents may test boundaries by making intimate inquiries about the counselor's marital status, whether or not he/she has children, and the job choices his or her children have taken. Such inquiries may be merely inquisitive and represent possible opportunities to learn more about the child. The motivations for these inquiries can be investigated without having to provide an answer. They may also wish to communicate with the counselor individually by messaging on social media and other channels.

The concept of therapeutic neutrality is essential and very helpful in navigating these circumstances. Therapeutic neutrality can be a useful guideline for navigating the counseling/psychotherapy process with a teenager. Neutrality does not imply that the mental health professional does not care for the child/adolescent or does not respond to the unfolding process emotionally. The counselor will not support or condemn the teenager, his or her parents, or their conduct, but will remain interested in understanding what they represent for the adolescent. Mental health professionals must recognize that therapy concerns with teenagers may extend beyond transference and countertransference and that adolescents' impressions of the counselor, as well as vice versa, can provide valuable information regarding the conflicts at hand.

AUTONOMY

The adolescent's ability to contribute to judgments based on comprehension and impartiality is becoming more widely recognized. There are many clinical and ethical reasons for adolescents to be involved in treatment decisions, including psychotherapy. The working partnership is reinforced when the adolescent believes he or she made an informed decision to pursue psychotherapy rather than having it imposed on him or her. In today's world, where adolescents are well-read and knowledgeable, they must be involved in treatment decisions affecting them when they have the insight and intelligence to decide rather than consent, which must be supplied by their parents. All decisions in adolescent psychotherapy must be made with parental views and sociocultural factors in mind.

CONFIDENTIALITY

The counselor working with teenagers has a strict duty to keep information about the adolescent and his or her family private.

These concepts also serve as the foundation for the adolescent's connection with the mental health professional concerned. Only by establishing trust and confidence can a therapeutic environment be formed. Within this place, the adolescent can feel safe enough to trust the freedom to divulge all without fear of being judged, retaliated against, or condemned. Especially in the Indian society, parental eagerness to know what is going on with the child/adolescent can sometimes put the counselor in difficulty. The "best-interest-of-the-child" doctrine helps in navigating these challenges.

POTENTIALLY HARMFUL BEHAVIORS

Using substances, sexual exploitation, suicidality, deliberate self-harm (DSH), and aggressive behaviors are few instances which can be really challenging when a counselor encounters them. The doctrine called "best interest of the child" is the vital guide in this situation. Taking the child on their side before the information is revealed to the authority concerned is very essential. Conveying in very simple terms how this move is in the child's best interest is crucial, though time consuming.

MEETING CLIENTS AT PUBLIC PLACES

Although public encounters are frequently surprising, some can be predicted and avoided. When a counselor is aware that an adolescent will be present at an event that he or she attends, the counselor may choose to avoid the event or discuss the anticipated interaction with the adolescent ahead of time. In general, counselors should emphasize to the teenager and his or her parents that, outside of the office, one will err on the side of not acknowledging them unless they begin an acknowledgment.

RESPONSIBILITIES AS A COUNSELOR TOWARD PARENTS/LEGAL GUARDIANS

Counselors, in accordance with current legal and custodial arrangements, inform parents and legal guardians about the function of counselors and the confidential nature of the counseling relationship. They are sensitive to the cultural diversity of families and respect parents'/guardians' fundamental rights and duties regarding the welfare of their children/charges under the law. Counselors work to create collaborative connections with parents/guardians as needed in order to effectively serve clients.

Finally, some counselors will work with the child and parents to create a "best interests" agreement. The counselor establishes the boundaries of secrecy in this agreement, and the children and parents leave the decision to reveal information completely with him or her. It is understood that confidentiality will be kept unless the counselor considers that the adolescent's health, welfare, or significant relationships are not being serviced in the best interests of the child. If any of these areas is badly harmed, the counselor uses his or her discretion to determine whether confidentiality should be violated. Again, a formal agreement can help to cement the deal between all parties.

CONCLUSION

Counselors work under legal and ethical mandates that are not intended to impede the process or cause problems for the counselor or client. Rather, most have stood the test of time and appear to clearly signify the values and intrinsic good of the finest counseling. Our field is anchored and built on the foundation of trust. Often, trust arises from doing the right thing rather than simply employing words and phrases that attract the client's attention. In circumstances, where the counselor is unsure about what to do, there are resources and preset mandates on which to rely.

Counselors must evaluate their professional code of ethics on a regular basis and update their ethical skills and knowledge through ongoing education in ethics and legal concerns. This training helps keep counselors up to date on new laws (including case laws). Many professional organizations give such training at conferences or through home study. Although client welfare and risk management must be carefully weighed when counseling children, there are significant benefits for the child, family, and, ultimately, our society's future.

DEDICATION

This chapter is dedicated to all children and adolescents who are and will continue being the best teachers in my life.

SUGGESTED READING

1. D'Souza R, De Sousa A. Ethical issues in psychotherapy with adolescents. Global Bioeth Enquiry. 2020;8:119.
2. Ministry of Women and Child Development. [online] Available from https://wcd.nic.in/sites/default/files/Protection%20of%20 Children% 20From%20Sexual%20Offences %20%28Amendment% 29% 20Act%2C%202019.pdf. [Last accessed September, 2024].
3. Sartor TA, McHenry B, McHenry J (Eds). Ethical and Legal Issues in Counseling Children and Adolescents. London: Routledge; 2016.
4. Sori CF, Hecker LL. Ethical and legal considerations when counseling children and families. In: Engaging Children in Family Therapy. London: Routledge; 2012. pp. 159-74.
5. UNICEF. What is the UNCRC? [online] Available from https://www.unicef.org.uk/what-we-do/un-convention-child-rights/ [Last accessed September, 2024].

11 CHAPTER

Behavior Modification Techniques

Indira MS, MKC Nair

INTRODUCTION

The term "behavior" may be interpreted broadly to include (1) overt responses—behaviors which may be observed like restless, pacing, fainting, nail biting, and quickened breathing, and (2) covert responses—emotions and implicit verbalizations. The behavioral approach has been misconceived to be only technique-oriented; teaching clients how to handle problems using manipulative techniques. Although techniques are used in the behavioral approach, the human aspect is never ignored and ethical considerations are strictly kept in mind.

HAPPINESS

Happiness is an outstanding characteristic of mental health, and it is an important prerequisite of good adjustment. Adjustment is a continuous process of satisfying one's desires and it involves many aspects of behavior. Erik Erikson considered adjustment as a lifelong process according to him, the basis of mental health was the mastery of crisis at successive life stages. Sigmund Freud described mental health as expressing oneself in love and in work. The well-adjusted person finds fulfilment in both these respects. Abraham Maslow evaluated the well-adjusted person in terms of self-actualization, clearly stressing the adjustment process. Human beings constantly seek expression of their potential, and those developing and utilizing their capacities to the fullest are said to be self-actualizing. Carl Rogers cited two dimensions of the adjustment process: openness to experience and trust in oneself.

BEHAVIOR MODEL

The behavior model is characterized by many assumptions, which differentiate it from the psychodynamic and humanistic models.

- Relative to the other methods of psychotherapy, behavior modification tends to concentrate on the behavior itself rather than on some presumed underlying cause.
- Assumes that maladaptive behaviors are to a large extent acquired through learning, in the same way that any behavior is acquired
- Assumes that learning principles can be extremely effective in modifying maladaptive behavior
- Involves setting specific goals
- Rejects classical trait theory
- Adopts the counselor's methods of treatment to the client's problem
- Focuses on the present rather than on the past
- Places great emphasis on observable and measurable responses and on obtaining empirical support for their various techniques.

BEHAVIOR COUNSELING

The common features as also in other types of counseling are as follows:

- Establishing a helping relationship
- Obtaining information about the client
- Carrying out suitable assessment procedures
- Carrying out the therapeutic process.

The initial focus should be on identifying the problems of the client and understanding them from his/her perspective. The next step would be to focus on helping the client acquire a broader, a more realistic alternate frame of reference or, in other words, to see the problems as they actually are and as others may view them—a new conceptualization of the problems. This should then lead to setting of goals for change, identifying target behaviors, and choosing problem management strategies. The counselor then supports the client on the various steps he/she takes to deal with the problem. It should be remembered that although the therapist often talks more and influences the session, the client is an active participant in both the assessment and interventions.

Steps in the Process of Behavior Counseling

- Selection of the target behavior that needs to be changed
- Establishment of baseline behavior through observation and recording
- Identification of the relationship between the target behavior and the factors that initiate or maintain them
- Application of reinforces as per agreement between the therapist and the client
- Recording of progress
- Reduction of external reinforces and moving to intrinsic reinforces and self-motivation.

Behavior is Maintained by Its Consequences

If the counselor wants to modify the behavior of the child, he/she needs to work on controlling the consequences rather than the behavior. All too often, we adults try to control the child's behavior directly through commands, manipulation, lectures, and other ineffective ways.

- If one wants the child to do something more often, increase the consequences that are rewarding the behavior, or provide some rewarding consequences.
- If one wants the child to stop doing something, look for the consequences that are rewarding the behavior and stop them.
- Punishment is the least effective way of controlling behavior.
- Behavior can be controlled through the proper use of punishment but made worse through improper use.
- When behavior is being extinguished by removing the rewards, expect the behavior to get worse temporarily.
- If one is not ready to remove cent percent of the rewards, do not do anything. It could make the behavior much worse than before.
- If the desired behavior never occurs, then reward behaviors that are similar or that can lead to the desired behavior.
- The timing of a reward or punishment is extremely important.
- Children will discriminate between people who use effective methods and those who do not, and will behave differently for each.

- Children are very adaptive and are able to do well even though one makes a lot of mistakes.

BEHAVIOR THERAPY

There are a number of behavior therapy techniques that are used to modify the behavior pattern or to change the undesirable/ maladjusted behaviors of individuals. In behavior modification, the maladaptive behavior is given more emphasis and assumes that maladaptive behaviors, to a large extent, are acquired through learning. Learning principles are used in modifying the maladaptive behavior. Behavior modification aims at modifying behavior by reinforcing acceptable behavior and suppressing undesirable behavior. The therapist employs any of the various techniques of reward and punishment including:

- Aversion therapy
- Desensitization
- Guided imagery.

The learning theory of Skinner and others is the basis for most behavior therapies. In Skinner's principle of extinction, a behavior pattern that is not reinforced or rewarded will be extinguished or rendered inoperative.

BEHAVIOR MODIFICATION

Behavior modification may deal with behaviors that are maladaptive in that they are obviously self-defeating. Behavior modification techniques that may be used in clinical, educational, and organizational settings areas follows:

- Relaxation
- Systematic desensitization (SD)
- Assertive training
- Modeling
- Operant conditioning
- Self-control procedures
- Aversive conditioning
- Cognitive behavior modification.

Relaxation Techniques

These are procedures that make an individual learn systematically to relax and make it a habit, so that tension is eliminated by bringing it under one's voluntary control. Tension may be experienced as psychological symptoms of inability to concentrate, poor memory, difficulty in making decisions, negative thinking, a feeling of threat, fatigue, or somatic symptoms like excessive sweating, palpitations, tensed muscles, shortness of breath, giddiness, tremors, flushed or pale face, and dry throat.

Jacobson's Progressive (Deep) Muscle Relaxation

This is based on the principle that muscle tension is somehow related to anxiety and an individual will experience a very marked and comforting reduction in felt anxiety if tense muscles are made loose and flaccid. A powerful and efficient method for effecting such a state of muscle relaxation involves the successive tensing and relaxing of voluntary muscles in an orderly progressive sequence until all the main muscle groups of the body are relaxed.

- Relaxation can be practiced either by lying flat on the back or by sitting comfortably in a reclining posture.
- *External environment:* The room should be dimly lit, noise free, and well ventilated.
- *Internal environment:* Relaxation should not be practiced after a heavy meal.
- The therapist supervises and facilitates the process while encouraging the client to go through the procedure himself/herself.

Autogenic Relaxation Training

In this method, the therapist teaches the client to engage in autosuggestion to the effect that his/her body is heavy and warm. The heaviness presumably leads to muscle flaccidity and warmth to vasodilatation, and both are associated with feelings of subjective relaxation. Other suggestions are with reference to heart rate, breathing rate, abdominal warmth, and cool feeling on the forehead.

Savasana

As the very term suggests, *savasana* is assuming the posture of a dead body or, in other words, lying flat on the back with absolutely no trace of motion either in the body or in the mind, as if the individual is dead.

Yoga Nidra

An extension of *savasana*, *yoga* refers to a system of exercise to free the self from the body, will, and mind, and *nidra* means sleep. This is a technique in which the individual, assuming the posture of sleep, practices a series of steps, giving more active role to the mind than to the body so as to introduce the state of relaxation in him/her.

Systematic Desensitization

Systematic desensitization (SD), developed by Joseph Wolpe, is a popular and effective method of treating anxiety, phobias, and excessive anger, aimed specifically at the alleviation of maladaptive anxiety. The technique involves the pairing of relaxation with imagined scenes depicting situations that the client has indicated, causing him/her to feel anxious. The therapist usually operates on the assumption that if the client is taught to experience relaxation rather than anxiety while imagining such scenes, and in the real-life situation, it will cause much less discomfort. SD is based on the principle of counterconditioning; that is, in this context, relaxation is substituted for anxiety. SD, in other words, is used for behavior that is negatively reinforced—reinforced by the successful avoidance of a painful situation which is harder to deal with.

The therapist after the interview with the client must decide whether the anxiety is rational or irrational. If it appears that the client's anxiety does not result from an objective lack of skills or from an objectively dangerous situation, SD may be an appropriate treatment.

Construction of Stimulus Hierarchy

Hierarchy is a graded series of situations or scenes that the client is likely to imagine while in a state of relaxation. A stimulus hierarchy consists of a graded series of events, all related to one particular theme, that evoke gradually increasing degrees of anxiety. This starts with a stimulation that elicits just a small amount of discomfort and ranging to those that provoke high discomfort.

Assertion Training

Assertion training refers to the behavior therapy procedure in which an individual is instructed, coached, trained, and supported in taking positive assertive action in situations (social skill training). Assertive behavior is the skill to seek, maintain, or enhance reinforcement in an interpersonal situation and is different from aggression. Lazarus suggested four response categories involved in assertive behavior:

1. Ability to initiate, continue, and successfully terminate conversations
2. Ability to say "no"
3. Ability to make request or ask for favors
4. Ability to express positive and negative feelings.

Procedure of Assertion Training

- *Step 1:* Identify the specific areas in which one is having difficulty.
- *Step 2:* Irrational ideas are dealt with by using cognitive restructuring methods like relaxation procedures.
- *Step 3:* The client is taught to use the right body posture and to adapt proper tone and volume of his/her voice according to the situation.
- *Step 4:* Various aspects of verbal communication also receive attention in the training:
    - Assertive talk which includes asserting one's rights and paying a compliment
    - Expressing feelings
    - Greeting others
    - Showing disagreements
    - Asking "why"
    - Talking about oneself
    - Rewarding others for compliments
    - Refusing to justify opinions to people who are in the habit of arguing

- *Step 5:* Role reversal can also be done with the trainer playing the part of the client.

Components of Social Skills Training

- *Behavioral rehearsal:* Provide for learning new behaviors and allow their practice in a safe environment.
- *Feedback:* Positive feedback is offered after each rehearsal.
- *Promoting:* Instructions/signals are used to prompt a response.
- *Model presentation:* Demonstrations help to improve the client's response.
- *Programming of change:* Establishing specific goals for each session
- *The use of homework assignments:* Assignment in the client's natural environment can be given once the skills are attained.
- *The use of logs during intervention:* A daily record of progress needs to be maintained.

Operant Conditioning Techniques

The procedure involves the selective use of reinforcement and punishment to change behavior in desired directions. Reinforcement refers to a sequence of events that increase the probability of a behavior occurring in the future. There are two kinds of reinforcement—positive and negative.

- *Reinforcement:* Positive stimulus presented following desirable behavior
- *Reinforcement:* Negative stimulus removed following desirable behavior
- *Punishment:* Negative stimulus presented following undesirable behavior
- *Punishment:* Positive stimulus removed following undesirable behavior

Cognitive Behavior Modification

Cognitive approaches to modifying behavior try to achieve changes in behavior by altering thought patterns, beliefs, attitudes, and opinions.

Self-instruction

The philosophy is that people can teach or coach themselves:

- Repeating helpful reminders to oneself to relax
- Interpreting problems differently
- Reminding oneself of helpful actions to take
- Remembering to self-reward.

Cognitive Therapy

Cognitive therapy is based on the notion that psychological problems result from faulty thinking. The goal of the therapy is to correct unreasonable thinking by the therapist taking an active role and doing most of the talking. Beck believed that almost all depression resulted from people's unrealistically negative views of themselves, the future, and the world. The cognitive therapist identifies these negative thoughts and replaces them with more realistic approaches, as they believe that if thinking is changed, attitudes and behavior will also change.

Rational Emotive Therapy

Rational emotive therapy is a form of therapy that helps people think rationally and eliminate their self-defeating emotional thoughts. It is assumed that people learn irrational and self-defeating prepositions in their youth. For example, some people may assume that life would be horrible if they are unpopular and as a result they limit and restrict themselves and are not willing to take chances. In rational emotive therapy (RET), the therapist would teach these people to re-examine their beliefs. RET is most appropriate for clients with above-average intelligence.

Behavioral Analysis Based on the *ABC* Model

ABC stands for:

- *A:* Antecedents
- *B:* Behavior
- *C:* Consequences

The three important steps in the assessment and clinical formulation while conducting behavior therapy are: (1) specification of problem behavior, (2) measurement of problem behavior, and (3) assessment of the function of the problem behavior.

Specification

Describe the behavior in question as precise as possible—onset, when, where, how, how different, how same, how it continues, how it ends, etc. There should be no subjective bias and idiosyncratic understanding of the behavior.

Measurement

Target behaviors are measured in terms of frequency, duration, intensity, and latency (the time that lapses between an important event and the onset of the behavior). Information can be collected from direct interview, self-report, parental interview and report, teacher report, rating scale, etc. Measurement is essential to decide whether:

- The behavior actually is a "problem behavior"
- Intervention is warranted
- It is important to evaluate the efficacy of behavior intervention.

Assessment of the Function

Identify the antecedents and consequences of the problem behavior. Information is collected from direct observation and interviews with the parent and child. There should be no subjective bias, no taking sides. Almost always, there should be consensus between the parent and the child regarding antecedent and consequences. Evaluation should be ongoing and can be updated with sessions if required. Along with these three steps, find out the strength and weakness of the individual, so that they can be included in the intervention model.

CONCLUSION

Behavior modification techniques are used to modify maladaptive and problem behaviors. Initially a baseline assessment of problem behavior is noted and then a behavior modification technique like operant conditioning, relaxation, systemic desensitization, cognitive behavior therapy or assertive communication technique is advised depending on the type of problem behavior. The assessment is repeated during follow up at regular intervals to objectively assess the improvement in behavior.

SUGGESTED READING

1. Behavior Modification Therapy for Struggling Adolescents. California: Aspen Youth Services; 2001.
2. Pfiffner LJ, Haack LM. Behavior management for school-aged children with ADHD. Child Adolesc Psychiatr Clin N Am. 2014;23:731-46.
3. Wolman BB. Dictionary of Behavioral Sciences. London: Van Nostrand Reinhold Company; 1989.

CHAPTER 12

Dialectical Behavior Therapy Principles in Counseling

Vinayak Koparde

INTRODUCTION

The field of psychotherapy has evolved over time significantly and so has its application on counseling. Starting from behavior therapy, then cognitive and most recently cognitive behavioral therapy (CBT) is used as an evidence-based approach. Dialectical behavior therapy (DBT) was conceptualized by Marsha Linehan while treating suicidal behavior in adults with borderline personality disorder (BPD). Over time, DBT has been used for adolescents struggling with behavioral and emotional dysregulation across the world due to mounting positive research findings. DBT for adolescents has been studied and used in suicidal ideation/behavior, nonsuicidal self-injury (NSSI), eating disorders, trichotillomania, externalizing disorders, and mood disorders, to name a few. While working with adolescents, various techniques of DBT are used in counseling.

THEORETICAL FOUNDATION OF DIALECTICAL BEHAVIOR THERAPY

Dialectical behavior therapy is a form of CBT with the inclusion of mindfulness and acceptance techniques. In other words, DBT not only operates on the principles of behavioral science at one end but also has components of dialectical philosophy with essence of Zen practice to a larger extent. DBT works on behavioral principles, where challenging behaviors are seen as learned behaviors. DBT model tries to change maladaptive behaviors in adolescents by identifying the triggers for these and trying to change the contingencies that maintain these behaviors in therapy. DBT works to reinforce adaptive behaviors and extinguish maladaptive ones by providing a validating environment with the therapist. Dialectical philosophy operates on the principle that the opposing views can be present in a person at the same time, which can result in conflict, and according to Linehan, DBT works to resolve this conflict by understanding and accepting this reality of opposite views.

DIALECTICAL BEHAVIOR THERAPY AS A MULTIMODAL THERAPY

Dialectical behavior therapy involves helping young people (YP) through individual therapy, skills training in groups, coaching YP over telephone, and consultation team meetings among therapists. The strategies of these multimodal therapies can be used while counseling adolescents having issues related to suicidal thoughts, self-harm, anger issues, eating difficulties, mood fluctuations, and several others. These strategies are discussed in subsequent sections.

Individual Therapy

Therapist works one-on-one with the YP to address goals and rules of treatment, identify and analyze problem-solving, and work on building skills to manage distressing emotions, such as anger, sadness, and frustration. YP are asked to keep a daily record of mood rating, problem behaviors displayed, and newer skills used to manage. These are analyzed in therapy and new healthy strategies are learned.

Dialectical Strategies

Dialectical strategies are central to DBT, and the therapist works with YP to change maladaptive thoughts or behavior. The therapist engages with YP by offering an alternative viewpoint about an event and then encouraging them to see how synthesis can be achieved among opposing views, thus promoting dialectical thinking and behavior. Some strategies described by Linehan are as follows:

- *Devil's advocate:* Synthesis can be achieved by the therapist arguing against a certain perspective to help the YP argue for it.
- *Use of metaphor:* Another engaging way using metaphors helps develop alternate views.
- *Making lemonade out of lemons:* Here, the therapist takes a problem in YP's life and tries to turn it into something positive.

Validation Strategies

Where a therapist accepting the young person and making her feel that their responses make sense within the context they are in goes on a long way.

Problem-solving Strategies

The therapist with YP understands and labels selected problem behavior, such as self-harm or aggression, and each behavior goes through *behavioral chain analysis*. This chain analysis initially identifies vulnerable situations YP were living in, then antecedent events, followed by thoughts generated, feelings and sensations experienced, and lastly behavior that led to the problem behavior, and consequences YP had to face. Then a *solution analysis* is carried out which identifies various points in the behavioral chain analysis that can interrupt the chain of events and prevent the problem behavior.

Group Skills Training

These are conducted weekly for 2–2.5 hours and focus on teaching new skills, i.e., mindfulness, distress tolerance, emotion regulation, and interpersonal effectiveness.

Mindfulness

Mindfulness skills are core to DBT, derived from Zen practice, and involve being in the present moment, doing one activity at a time, with complete attention and acceptance. There are two parts that need to be taught: First, awareness where YP are coached to focus on the present moment, paying attention to whatever the YP are doing—reading, talking, walking, and listening to songs. The second part is acceptance, where YP learn to just be aware of their experience and not judge it. So if the YP are feeling anxious, they try to simply accept it first. Then if the YP notice that they are not interested, they try to just acknowledge it. One example that can help YP to understand mindfulness better is the *monkey mind analogy*, which states that the mind is like a monkey. It goes on jumping from place to place, easily distracted and trying to see different things, and difficult to hold. This helps YP understand their own experience of mind being restless and difficulties arising while practicing mindfulness.

Mindfulness practices that can be taught to YP are counting breaths, observing an object in their environment or a sound, and focusing on a thought without judging it. The YP are coached to select an activity to focus on, then concentrate on that activity, and keep a note on when attention wanders. In therapy, YP learn to gently bring back the attention through practice many times.

Distress Tolerance

Skills are taught to YP to control impulses, distract, and self-soothe whenever they are faced with a challenging situation without resorting to problem behavior. Examining cost and benefit of problem behavior is one such strategy for the YP to discuss in therapy. Other strategies are described using the acronym RESISTT in **Table 1**.

TABLE 1: Distress tolerance skills—RESISTT.

R	*R*eframe the problem by giving a different perspective to the problem
E	*E*ngage mindfully in an activity
S	Do something for *S*omeone else, e.g., visiting a friend who needs help, spending time to cook, or helping for a family member
I	*I*ntense sensations—YP to distract the mind from painful emotions can inflict intense sensations. YP can do these things to distract their mind from a crisis situation: • Wash face or take a cold-water shower • Put a rubber band on wrist and intermittently snap it, so that mild painful sensation will distract the mind • Hold or chew ice cubes • Go out of the situation; walk some distance
S	*S*hut it out
T	*T*hink neutral *T*houghts • Say your favorite prayer • Sing or listen to your favorite song • Tell the names of objects around you, e.g., chair, book, photo, fan, and so on • Repeat a mantra, such as "Calm down" or "Shanti"
T	*T*ake a break

Emotion Regulation

One of the common concerns in adolescents is their inability to control emotional expressions due to ongoing maturation of the brain. Teaching YP skills of emotional regulation starts with the identification of various emotions they express in a moment, then describing them, and finally determining whether their emotional expression is justified in the current circumstance. YP are coached in regulating emotions by several strategies, such as self-validation, increasing positive emotions by engaging in acceptable pleasurable activities, acting opposite to their emotion, and learning problem-solving skills.

Self-validation: Accepting emotions is one important skill YP learn through DBT. YP commonly invalidate their feelings/emotions and judge negatively for their inability to regulate emotions. Self-validation is practiced in three levels of *acknowledging*, where they simply acknowledge the presence of the emotion without judging it; *allowing* oneself to feel emotion that it is okay to feel unhappy; and finally having an *understanding* of the whole situation and emotions, for example, YP going through a situation reflecting as "It makes sense that I feel sad, as I find difficulty in managing my emotions and all that as a result of problems going in my life". YP can learn to manage their emotions using the acronym *WATCH* described in **Table 2**.

TABLE 2: Self-validation skills—WATCH.

W	*W*atch your emotions. Feel physical sensations, observe thoughts or memories or images that accompany the emotions
A	*A*void knee-jerk reaction in an incident and think that it is just an emotion that does not require any reaction
T	*T*hink that overwhelming emotional experience as a wave and understand that it will have to recede on its own
C	*C*hoose to let yourself experience the emotion which will help in long term
H	*H*elpers—see emotions as your helpers, which make you learn important things

Other strategies that can be useful in managing emotions are:

- Mindfulness to let go negative emotions
- Increasing positive experiences
- Increasing pleasurable activities—time with pets, play with children, and listen to music
- *Being effective:* Analyzing when they have done something they later regretted and working on preventing such reactions
- *The half-smile:* There is a saying: "Sometimes your joy is the source of your smile, but sometimes your smile can be the source of your joy". Putting on a half-smile is a simple DBT skill where YP are coached to slightly turn up the corners of their mouth. This half-smile expression will help increase positive emotions.

Interpersonal Effectiveness

Interpersonal effectiveness teaches assertiveness skills to maintain positive relationships and self-respect. Communication style plays an important role in relationships. Counselors can develop assertiveness using the following skills in YP:

- Help decide on priorities—improving a relationship
- YP can make requests in a gentle way, which will not harm relationships, by describing the situation and related thoughts and feelings.
- Negotiate to come to a point of agreement
- Obtaining information—asking for more information about an issue
- Learning to say No in gentle manner

Telephone Coaching Calls

Young people can call the therapist when experiencing self-harm to seek help on implementing and choosing a DBT skill to cope with mental distress. They can call therapist for a short duration, usually 5–15 minutes, to get feedback about the problem and see which skill can best be used. Counselors can use this strategy effectively to support YP and monitor risk issues.

Therapist Team Meetings

These consultation meetings among therapists lasting 1–2 hours help in reflection of ongoing problems encountered in therapy, interaction with the YP, and understanding blocks that may be affecting progress in therapy. Counselors having a group and supervision will help immensely to understand problems and manage them while working with YP.

The process of helping adolescents going through a tough time can be a challenging task for a therapist. Making use of DBT principles with its multimodal strategies can help a counselor feel confident in this process. Even though manualized DBT is an intensive, time, and skilled process that therapists learn after years of practice and supervision, being aware of the strategies and willing to use them should build the skill set of counselors. Counselors understanding and using DBT skills, such as dialectical strategies, mindfulness, distress tolerance skills, and emotion regulation skills, will empower them in managing adolescents going through a range of maladaptive behaviors.

CONCLUSION

Dialectical philosophy operates on the principle that opposing views can be present in a person at the same time which can result in conflict, and resolving this conflict in counselling helps reduce symptoms. DBT is also conceptualized as a form of CBT with inclusion of mindfulness and acceptance techniques. It has multi-modal therapy approach involving individual therapy, group therapy, telephone based coaching and team meetings among therapists. Adolescent maladaptive behaviours such as self-harm or aggression are helped in counselling using behavioral chain analysis and solution analysis. Distress tolerance and emotion regulation skills are learnt by adolescent in counselling based on DBT principles.

SUGGESTED READING

1. Asarnow JR, Berk MS, Bedics J, Adrian M, Gallop R, Cohen J, et al. Dialectical behavior therapy for suicidal self-harming youth: emotion

regulation, mechanisms, and mediators. J Am Acad Child Adolesc Psychiatry. 2021;60(9):1105-15.e4.

2. Koerner K. Doing Dialectical Behavior Therapy: A Practical Guide. New York: Guilford Press; 2011.
3. Kothgassner OD, Goreis A, Robinson K, Huscsava MM, Schmahl C, Plener PL. Efficacy of dialectical behavior therapy for adolescent self-harm and suicidal ideation: a systematic review and meta-analysis. Psychol Med. 2021;51(7):1057-67.
4. Linehan MM, Heard H, Clarkin J, Marziali E, Munroe-Blum H. Dialectical Behavior Therapy for Borderline Personality Disorder. New York: Guilford Press; 1993.
5. MacPherson HA, Cheavens JS, Fristad MA. Dialectical behavior therapy for adolescents: theory, treatment adaptations, and empirical outcomes. Clin Child Fam Psychol Rev. 2013;16:59-80.
6. van Dijk S. DBT Made Simple: A Step-By-Step Guide to Dialectical Behavior Therapy. Oakland: New Harbinger Publications; 2013.

13 CHAPTER

Cognitive Behavior Therapy Principles in Counseling

Swati Ghate, Shubhada Khirwadkar

INTRODUCTION

Cognitive behavioral therapy (CBT), which is an umbrella term for psychotherapies using cognitive and behavioral components, was conceptualized and popularized by Dr Aron Beck and Dr Albert Ellis. CBT and rational emotive behavior therapy (REBT), the main constituents therein, are scientifically proven psychotherapeutic methods that aim to reduce psychological distress and dysfunction caused by a variety of reasons, including psychopathologies. They explore and address the interplay of a client's thoughts, feelings, and behaviors responsible for their mental framework and conduct. We shall discuss the principles of Beck's CBT in this chapter.

Unlike preachy counseling that adolescents dislike, CBT believes in the rationalization of thoughts and structured organization of behaviors in an adolescent-friendly manner. Since adolescents' age group has a significantly high incidence of mental and behavioral issues, amounting to about one in five, principles of CBT prove to be a very useful tool to help many troubled teens.

Cognitive behavioral therapy is a systematic and methodical approach. Its principles ensure that it is optimally scientific, logical, practical, and yet retains the human touch.

Let us see how the CBT principles are put to use in the counseling sessions.

PRINCIPLE OF COLLABORATIVE EMPIRICISM

This involves establishing a therapeutic alliance between the mental health professional and the client. It ensures an agreement between both the parties to move further as a team. The adolescent has to have an insight and should feel the need to seek professional support to sort out his issues. But this is good enough only to bring him to the therapist's office. How he is received there and his experience in the initial session would decide whether he would feel like continuing the sessions. Hence, his commitment to cooperation and compliance, which are very necessary for a fruitful outcome of the therapy, is majorly decided by the therapist's adolescent-friendly approach and dealing.

The therapist should, therefore, empower himself with adolescent-specific counseling and communication skills. The first impression of a warm, gentle, and confident therapist who treats the adolescent with respect goes a long way in building rapport between the two. The adolescent should always be greeted, and some casual icebreaking conversation on his area of interest helps him open up. Active listening with undivided attention is something that teens look for. The therapist should possess and exhibit genuine interest in the client's problem. He should be empathetic and strictly avoid passing judgmental remarks. He should take a stand that whatever the client is going through, his feelings, behavior, and the way he expresses himself (e.g., with tears in his eyes and taking too long to answer) is completely understandable.

This helps making a team that works toward a defined goal as CBT expects active involvement and participation from the client, including doing home assignments and experiments.

PRINCIPLE OF HERE AND NOW

Cognitive behavioral therapy focuses on the present distress faced by clients, unlike psychoanalytical therapies, which emphasize on the past experiences. The therapist is interested in identifying the current problems, their severity, and their priority for the client. Hence, as the client narrates his version, the therapist encourages him to elaborate yet stick to the present. He intermittently paraphrase the narration in his own words and ensure that both of them are on the same page. He then summarizes the whole story and makes a crisp gist of it. This enables the client to exactly define his problems and arrange them pointwise.

For example: After listening to all that the adolescent narrated regarding his anger outbursts and fights with his father, the therapist said,

"So, it appears that you are unhappy with your father because he expects you to obey all his rules without allowing you to voice your opinion. This makes you feel being treated like a child and insulted".

This helps the client set his exact goals and prioritize them in a hierarchical manner.

The therapist then facilitates him in setting SMART (specific, measurable, achievable, rewarding, time-bound) goals.

COGNITIVE PRINCIPLES

Through this principle, CBT goes beyond emotions of the client and touches the higher mental abilities such as thought monitoring, rationalizing, mindfully reshaping the thoughts, and then testing and executing them. For this, clients are empowered with the core ideas on which the therapeutic intervention is based.

Cognitive Triad of Thoughts, Emotions, and Behavior

Cognitive behavioral therapy believes that in response to an experience (which could be an event or a thought in itself), we generate a variety of automatic thoughts. Depending on these thoughts, emotions of different shades arise in our minds **(Fig. 1)**.

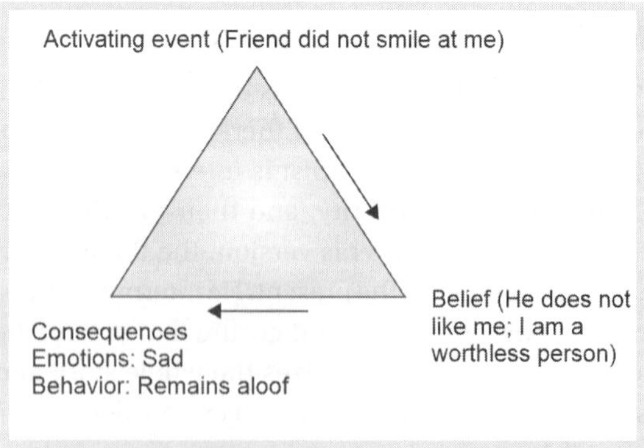

Fig. 1: ABC model.

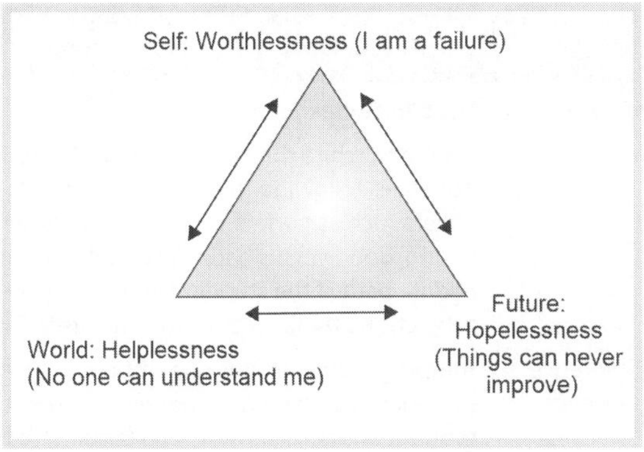

Fig. 2: Negative cognitive triad.

They could be positive or negative. These thoughts and emotions are the guiding agents that dictate our actions. If the thoughts are positive, we feel good and engage in productive, meaningful behaviors whereas if the thoughts generated are negative, we land in a negative state of mind and feel depressed, anxious, angry, etc. This makes us indulge in behaviors that are nonproductive or even harmful to self or others.

The negative cognitive triad comprises negative thoughts about oneself, the surrounding world, and/or the future. "I am a worthless person", "No one bothers for me", "Things will go wrong", and similar thoughts abound in a person, which makes him feel worthless, helpless, and hopeless **(Fig. 2)**. This state of mind reflects in his behaviors such as not caring for self, not mixing with people, and shunning away from making efforts.

These unhealthy unproductive behaviors further set the cycle of another negativity and escalate the situation.

Schemas and Erroneous Thoughts

The automatic thoughts are believed to arise out of "schemas" and cognitive errors.

Schemas are the impressions and mental images about issues surrounding us which we have gathered and carved over the years. They are maladaptive underlying assumptions. For example, an

TABLE 1: Cognitive errors: Types of erroneous thinking patterns and their explanations.

Cognitive error	***Description/examples***
Dichotomous thinking	Black and white thinking, display of extreme polarities, following the "all or none law". Extreme beliefs such as perfect versus useless, exact versus wrong, good versus bad, and unable to take a middle path. If the student fails once in one of the subjects, he thinks, "I am a total failure"
Arbitrary inference	Jumping to big conclusions without substantial evidence. If a friend does not give a smile, the thought arises, "Our friendship is going to break"
Selective abstraction	Filtering the good and focusing only on the not-so-good. A girl who has an overall good personality gets stuck on her short thin hair that she dislikes
Personalization	Pulling the onus on oneself without any convincing proof for the same. "It is me who has made her sad"
Future telling	Harboring negative thoughts about future without any justification. "I will never get a job"
Overgeneralization	Painting the entire picture dark, relying on just a small aspect of the whole. If the teacher scolds for a particular reason, the student thinks "I can never make my teacher happy"

adolescent girl might have a schema that beauty equates to thinness because she might have seen her dolls and actresses, models as thin-shaped. So if she puts on weight, she generates an automatic thought that "I am not beautiful", which makes her sad. Identifying and addressing such troubleshooter schemas form a part of CBT.

Cognitive errors are the fallacies in the mental processes that generate incorrect, illogical, faulty, and erroneous thoughts. Some important erroneous ways of thinking that cause distress are listed along with their explanatory descriptions in **Table 1**.

Cognitive Techniques

Cognitive behavioral therapy works on empowering the client to restructure his thoughts. Hence, first, all the basics of the abovementioned working principles are taught to the client. He is made well-versed with the concepts of cognitive triad, the maladaptive thoughts, and the cognitive errors.

- Cognitive techniques are first tried in the clinical setting and then given as homework. The client is encouraged to identify the automatic maladaptive thoughts and the event eliciting the thoughts. The underlying schemas and the erroneous beliefs are then found out. For example:
  - *A: Activating event:* Father scolds
  - *B: Belief/schema:* Fathers are disciplinarians and mothers are soft.
  - *C: Consequence:*
    - *Automatic thought:* My father is always angry with me.
    - *Cognitive error:* Overgeneralization
    - *Emotion:* Angry, sad
    - *Behavior:* Shouting, crying
- The next step is to test these thoughts for their reality, correctness, and logic, by eliciting the cognitive errors. The idea is to make the client realize that the trouble lies in the way he frames his self-talk and not so much in the situation, which he blame.

  Testing the automatic thought:
  - The client is asked to justify his statement.
  - Is father "always" angry? Does he not love you or care for you?
  - Can you list some good things he did for you last week?

  During this exercise, the client realizes that it is he who needs to change and gets a feeling of control over the situation. This arises hope in him and he starts looking for the addressal of his problems more optimistically. He also become more compliant if this stage is successfully achieved.
- *Reconstruction of the thought:*
  - The client is encouraged to reframe the thought to make it more rational, more logical, and less disturbing.
  - "My father is 'at times' angry with me".

This little change in perspective makes the client feel better, less angry, less sad, and hopeful of addressing the interpersonal relationship positively.

BEHAVIORAL PRINCIPLES

Cognitive behavioral therapy employs many practical techniques that the client is required to follow religiously. These activities are helpful for motivating the patient and engaging him meaningfully. These behaviors then turn into the events that generate positivity in his thoughts. Further, the behavioral activities come in handy as objective and observable accounts of the progress of CBT.

Behavioral techniques:

- *Mastery and pleasure tasks:* The client is asked to engage in activities he is good at and he derives pleasure from such as dancing and playing with pets. This makes him compliant and initiates positivity.
- *Activity scheduling and monitoring:* Organizing the day with the therapist and keeping a record of his activities helps the client stay motivated.
- *Hypothesis testing:* Here, the client is asked to write down the feared hypothesis and test it practically.

  "My boyfriend will laugh at me because I am fat". If a girl is carrying this hypothesis, she is encouraged to meet her boyfriend and observe the reaction and record it.
- *Record keeping:* Therapeutic journaling/mood monitoring/diary writing/allotting a specified "worry time".
- *Distraction:* Using a rubber band around the wrist and flicking it when the negative thoughts pop up are enough to distract the person.
- *Imagery technique:* Imagining happy outcomes and revisiting happy moments.

PRINCIPLE OF A STRUCTURED APPROACH

Cognitive behavioral therapy is time-bound and structured educating and helping technique. It aims at empowering the client to be his own therapist. It grants the powerful tools of reconstruction of thoughts and self-monitoring to the client, which he can use throughout his life, for multitudes of problems. Thus, it fosters his overall mental health.

Using these principles of CBT, either individually or in groups, one can help normative adolescents to make themselves emotionally more stable and functionally more competent. It is a very useful psychotherapeutic technique for anxiety, post-traumatic stress disorder (PTSD), obsessive-compulsive disorder (OCD), depression, relationship issues, body image distortion, and myriad of problems in adolescents as well as adults. A systematic plan of 6–12 sessions with or without medications suffices most of the patients with mild mental disorders.

CONCLUSION

CBT is based on the premise that thoughts, emotions and actions are interlinked.

It is a structured and evidence based psychotherapeutic technique for many psychopathologies.

Clients can be empowered to bring about positive change in their state of mind by systematically addressing their thoughts and actions.

SUGGESTED READING

1. Bhattacharya L, Chaudari B, Saldanha D, Menon P. Cognitive behavior therapy. Med J DY Patil Univ. 2013;6(2):132-8.
2. Halder S, Mahato AK. Cognitive behavior therapy for children and adolescents: challenges and gaps in practice. Indian J Psychol Med. 2019;41:279-83.
3. Sitaraman S, Ghate S. Cognitive behaviour therapy. In: Gupta BD, Maheshwari RK, Agrawal P, Aroroa AK, Purohit A, Choudhary SR (Eds). Behavioral Disorders in Children. New Delhi: Jaypee Brothers Medical Publishers; 2023.
4. Spirito A, Esposito-Smythers C, Wolff J, Uhl K. Cognitive-behavioral therapy for adolescent depression and suicidality. Child Adolesc Psychiatr Clin N Am. 2011;20:191-204.
5. Teater B. Cognitive behavioural therapy. In: Davies M (Ed). The Blackwell Companion to Social Work, 4th edition. Hoboken: Wiley-Blackwell; 2013.

14 CHAPTER

Strengths-based Counseling

Sreyoshi Ghosh

INTRODUCTION

Strengths-based counseling is an approach that focuses on identifying an individual's strengths as opposed to their weaknesses and how they have used their strengths to overcome difficult life circumstances. It is an approach that seeks to empower rather than pathologize a person seeking help. It is not directed by the clinician's agenda and what he or she feels is good for the client. Rather, it is collaborative and client-centric.

EVOLUTION OF THE CONCEPT

The traditional medical approach often focuses on addressing deficits and obstacles without always considering a child's existing strengths, resources, or environment that could be utilized in designing treatment plans. In the 1990s, Martin Seligman advocated for a shift in perspective toward "positive psychology", which highlights human strengths, virtues, and well-being.

Following this, Donald O Clifton, often referred to as "the father of strengths-based therapy", suggested that individuals can achieve greater success when efforts are directed toward reinforcing their strengths rather than dwelling on weaknesses. Helping adolescents recognize and utilize their strengths can foster hope and confidence in their ability to overcome challenges.

RATIONALE FOR A STRENGTHS-BASED APPROACH

It has been well supported by research that regardless of the type of counseling approach, certain factors that are transtheoretical are predictive of outcome. Of these, the quality of the rapport between the clinician and the patient is considered extremely important.

Thus, if developing rapport is directly linked to treatment efficacy, then an interview format that fosters hope, optimism, and agency may better facilitate this process. Schlechter et al. proposed a "positive assessment" that elicits information about the patient's well-being and strengths at the very outset. Although the traditional assessment format is designed to rapidly elicit problems and deficits, this strategy may inhibit the development of rapport, thereby potentially causing the client to drop out of treatment. Discussing the patient's strengths and well-being is more likely to encourage trust, hope, and a desire to change.

MAJOR THEORETICAL FRAMEWORKS OF COUNSELING THAT INCORPORATE A STRENGTHS-BASED APPROACH

Solution-focused therapy: The primary emphasis of solution-focused therapy has been to find solutions to clients' issues rather than focusing on their problems. Two counseling techniques that the strength-based model borrows from solution-focused therapy are the miracle question and the exception situation. The miracle question asks the client to imagine and discuss a possible world where problems are removed and issues addressed. The question may take various forms, such as asking the client, "Assume that when you wake up in the morning your problem has been solved. What is the first thing that you notice is different?" Or, "Assume your problem is gone. What does this mean to you?" The answers provided offer insights to the client while helping to define the goals for treatment.

The exception question operates on the premise that there were moments in clients' lives when issues were not apparent. Therapists using a solution-focused approach pose exception questions to direct clients' thoughts to occasions when the problem was not present. These exceptions highlight instances when the problem could have arisen but did not. Therapists then inquire about the necessary conditions for these exceptions to happen more frequently.

Narrative therapy: Narrative therapists help clients retell their life stories in a way that clients recall their strengths in dealing with problems rather than their weaknesses. For example, if clients present their story through the lens of being a victim of their circumstances, the clinician can invite them to recognize and acknowledge actions, intentions, and personal qualities that contradict the dominant themes of victimization and helplessness in their story.

Existential therapy/logotherapy: Viktor Frankl's logotherapy forms a cornerstone for strengths-based counseling, with its emphasis on the search to find meaning out of adversity.

LOOKING AT CLINICAL ASSESSMENT THROUGH A STRENGTH-BASED LENS

Strength-based assessment has been defined as the "measurement of those emotional and behavioral skills, competencies, and characteristics that create a sense of personal accomplishment; contribute to satisfying relationships with family members, peers, and adults; enhance one's ability to deal with adversity and stress; and promote one's personal, social, and academic development". While strength-based counselors prioritize finding solutions, they also need to invest time in gaining a thorough understanding of clients' perspectives on their issues during the assessment stage. Therefore, it is essential for the clinician to encourage clients to articulate their understanding of their problems, their reasons for believing why the problems exist, the behaviors or situations that pose the greatest challenges, and the resulting consequences of these problems. Selekman offers more examples of critical problem-finding questions that strength-based therapists might ask clients: "If there were one question that you were just dying to ask me about your problems, what would that question be?", "How can I be most helpful to you?", "What's your theory about why you have this problem?", and "If there were one question that you were hoping I would ask you, what would that question be?"

CONCLUSION

Strengths-based intervention prioritizes the positive attributes of patients that contribute to their well-being and complements the traditional medical approach to treating illnesses. This method operates under the belief that every individual has distinct aspirations and possesses internal strengths and external support systems to attain them. Its goal is to foster patients' sense of hope by enhancing their connections with themselves, family, therapy networks, community, and cultural roots. Integrating strengths-based intervention into conventional practice offers a comprehensive treatment strategy that cultivates optimism for the recovery of children and adolescents experiencing behavioral, emotional, and lifestyle challenges.

SUGGESTED READING

1. Buckingham M, Clifton DO. Now, Discover your Strengths. New York: Free Press; 2001.
2. Epstein MH. The behavioral and emotional rating scale: a strength-based approach to assessment. Diagnostique. 2000;25(3):249-56.
3. Frankl VE. Man's Search for Meaning: An Introduction to Logotherapy. New York: Washington Square Press; 1963.
4. Schlechter AD, O'Brien KH, Stewart C. The positive assessment: a model for integrating well-being and strengths-based approaches into the child and adolescent psychiatry clinical evaluation. Child Adolesc Psychiatr Clin N Am. 2019;28(2):157-69.
5. Selekman MD. Solution-Focused Therapy with Children: Harnessing Family Strengths for Systemic Change. New York: Guilford Press; 1997.
6. Seligman ME, Steen TA, Park N, Peterson C. Positive psychology progress: empirical validation of interventions. Am Psychol. 2005;60(5):410-21.
7. Smith EJ. The strength-based counseling model. Couns Psychol. 2006;34(1):13-79.
8. Strong T, Pyle NR. Constructing a conversational "miracle": examining the "miracle question" as it is used in therapeutic dialogue. J Constr Psychol. 2009;22(4):328-53.
9. White M, Epston D. Narrative Means to Therapeutic Ends. New York: WW Norton; 1990.

15 CHAPTER

Motivational Interviewing

Shubhada Khirwadkar, Swati Ghate

INTRODUCTION

In this chapter, we delve into motivational interviewing (MI), a counseling approach by Miller and Rollnick. Tailored for adolescents navigating the tumultuous journey of self-discovery, MI embraces a person-centered, collaborative method, rooted in humanistic psychology (Carl Rogers). Addressing the challenges of ambivalence and resistance, MI empowers individuals to uncover their intrinsic motivation, fostering sustainable positive change during the pivotal phase of adolescence.

DEFINITION

Motivational interviewing is a collaborative, goal-oriented style of communication, with particular attention to the language of change, designed to strengthen personal motivation for and commitment to a specific goal by eliciting and exploring the person's own reasons for change within an atmosphere of acceptance and compassion (Miller).

Imagine a therapist sitting across a hesitant adolescent, a chasm of uncertainty separating them. The air is thick with ambivalence and resistance, with a faint desire for change. The stage is thus set when the art of MI unfolds and conversations become a catalyst for change.

This chapter describes the spirit, core principles, essential steps, and practical skills of MI to engage, inspire, and guide young individuals.

THEORETICAL BACKGROUND

Adolescents, often brought to clinics by caregivers, may lack awareness of their detrimental behaviors and resist change.

TABLE 1: Stages of change.

Stage of change	*Description*
Precontemplation	Not realizing cons of a behavior, no consideration of change in future
Contemplation	Intending to make a healthier change in behavior, could be in two minds
Preparation	Determination and planning to take few steps
Action	Executing the plan to bring about change
Maintenance	Stabilizing the change in behavior, avoiding relapse

Prochaska and DiClemente's transtheoretical model defines stages of change, guiding nuanced counseling approaches based on individuals' readiness within the continuum. The five stages of change are delineated in **Table 1**.

Motivational interviewing delicately identifies individuals' stages, avoiding judgment and labels. Unlike structured therapies such as cognitive behavior therapy (CBT), MI suits those who are less self-efficacious. It refrains from being prescriptive, focusing on exploring and reinforcing intrinsic motivation, respecting clients' autonomy without skill building or didactic information sharing.

SPIRIT OF MOTIVATIONAL INTERVIEWING

Collaboration: In MI, collaboration is paramount. The counselor establishes a partnership, positioning the client as an expert in their values and goals. Acting as a facilitator, not a guide, the counselor empowers the client to navigate their issues.

Acceptance: Rooted in unconditional positive regard, MI fosters an environment of acceptance. The interviewer communicates the client's inherent worth and importance, expressing empathy. Acknowledging the client's efforts, MI supports complete autonomy in deciding when and how the behavioral change occurs.

Compassion: MI embodies kindness and consideration. The counselor promotes the client's welfare with gentleness, avoiding criticism and consciously cultivating a supportive atmosphere.

Evocation: MI believes in the client's strength and capacity to change. The counselor, adopting a noncorrective stance, uses open-ended questions to help the client articulate values and goals, revealing discrepancies therein and motivating change.

CORE PRINCIPLES OF MOTIVATIONAL INTERVIEWING

Express empathy: Central to MI is the principle of expressing empathy. The counselor must demonstrate a profound understanding and unconditional acceptance of adolescents' thoughts and feelings. Utilization of nonverbal cues such as eye contact, nodding, and body language, along with reflective listening and naming specific emotions, fosters rapport and builds trust. Seeking permission ensures a safe space for adolescents to open up freely.

Develop discrepancy: MI emphasizes that change arises from recognizing discrepancies between current behavior and personal goals. Rather than dictating issues, the counselor guides adolescents in identifying inconsistencies; for instance, acknowledging the impact of incomplete coursework on future goals or recognizing the health risks of smoking. Allowing adolescents to present their own reasons for change promotes self-discovery and commitment.

Avoid argumentation: Counterproductive to MI is direct argumentation and persuasion. The counselor refrains from imposing solutions, as it leads to resistance. MI asserts that effective and lasting behavior change originates from adolescents becoming the architects of their own solutions.

Rolling with resistance: Acknowledging ambivalence, MI advocates understanding and accepting where the adolescent stands. Instead of being pushy, the counselor respects the client's pace and is comfortable with silence, allowing the client to talk more than the clinician and giving them time to make decisions. This approach recognizes that effective change often stems from the client's own internal resolution.

Support self-efficacy: MI nurtures self-efficacy, the belief in one's ability to accomplish tasks. Emphasizing the slow, gradual nature of change and highlighting past successes and acquired skills, it instills confidence in the client. Encouraging adolescents to identify benefits and challenges in achieving goals reinforces their self-efficacy.

SKILLS OF MOTIVATIONAL INTERVIEWING

"OARS" is an apt acronym for skills which help navigate a motivational interview.

Open-ended questions: Central to MI, open-ended questions guide the counselor in exploring and evoking detailed responses from the client. Rather than closed queries such as "You agree that smoking is bad for health?," open-ended questions such as "Can you tell me about the impact of smoking on your life?" delve into the patterns of any problematic behavior, understanding its antecedents, triggers, and consequences. Some more examples of open questions could be as follows:

- Help me understand _____?
- How would you like things to be different?
- When would you be most likely to _____?
- What do you think you will lose if you give up _____?
- What have you tried before to make a change?
- What do you want to do next?

Affirmations: Affirmations in MI express genuine appreciation for the client's strengths and abilities. Carefully used, they reinforce positive aspects. For instance, "I really appreciate your being so honest with me!" These affirmations, when genuine, sincere, and sparingly applied, contribute to a supportive environment.

Reflections: Reflective listening involves warm, nonjudgmental restatements or enhancements of the client's narrative. Paraphrasing ensures precise understanding of the situation by the counselor and encourages clients who find it challenging to verbalize thoughts or emotions. In the context of an adolescent addressing problematic drinking and concerns about missing classes, a reflective response might be, "You're disappointed and upset when you miss out on things due to your drinking".

TABLE 2: Skills of motivational interviewing (MI).

Skill of MI	*Application*
Open-ended questions	Explore impact of behavior, avoid closed judgments
Affirmations	Genuinely, sincerely, and sparingly used for authenticity
Reflective listening	Nonjudgmental statements that help adolescents to express implicit emotions
Summarizing	Utilized during exploration, emphasizes key aspects of a conversation fostering comprehensive understanding

Summarizing: Summaries in MI gather the client's statements regarding thoughts and feelings. For example, "This behavior has become a cause of your underperformance in school and sports, which you wish to improve". Summarizing helps consolidate the client's perspective and emphasizes key points during the discussion.

The skills and their application are summarized in **Table 2**.

In MI sessions, the counselor navigates the challenges of behavior change by respectfully discussing possibilities for healthier behaviors. These discussions align with the client's goals and values, emphasizing autonomy and seeking permission before exploring alternative approaches. Through OARS (open-ended questions, affirmations, reflective listening, and summarizing), MI provides a structured approach to reinforce effective communication, promoting a positive change in adolescents.

The process of MI is often considered to be of step ladder pattern, which is sequential as well as recursive **(Fig. 1)**. The steps such as engaging a client, focusing on goals and values, evoking statements of intrinsic motivation to change, and exploring ways to execute the plans occur in a sequence in the flow of conversation. However, if at any step the counselor finds resistance or distraction, he can come back to the previous step and put in his efforts at that step to move ahead in the counseling process. The following stepwise approach is used to address the process of change.

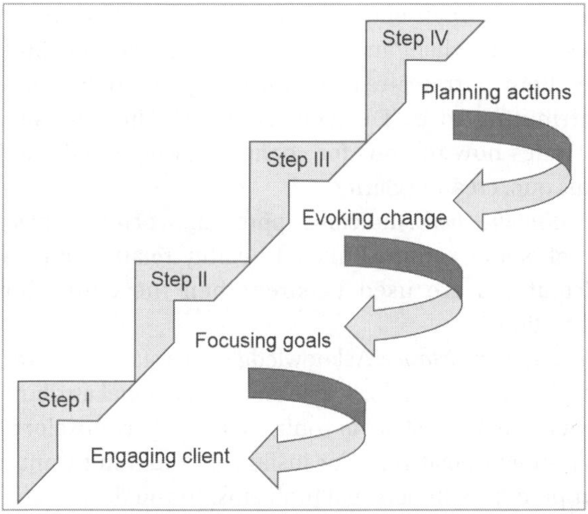

Fig. 1: Stepwise, recursive model of motivational interviewing (MI).

STEPS IN THE PROCESS OF MOTIVATIONAL INTERVIEWING

Step 1: Building Motivation for Change

In this crucial step, the focus shifts from the current state to the desired change, employing the following strategic approaches:

1. *Evoking self-motivational statements:* Clients are prompted to articulate what changes they envision for a better life. Nonaccusatory and nonthreatening questions such as "What do you like about drinking?" and "What worries you about drinking?" facilitate self-reflection. Authoritarian statements are avoided to empower the client's self-expression.
2. *Listening with empathy:* The counselor practices patient and attentive listening, reframing both content and emotions without judgment or confrontation. Rather than offering advice, the counselor objectively reflects the client's expressions. For instance, if a client expresses concern about quitting drinking due to friends, the counselor empathetically acknowledges, "It is hard for you to see yourself living without alcohol".

3. *Questioning:* Open-ended questions are used to explore various aspects of the client and the problem without providing advice. The client narrates reasons for or against behavior change, contributing to a "Decision Balance". The counselor then illustrates how reasons for change outweigh maintaining the status quo, creating clarity.
4. *Affirming the client:* Judicious appreciation of the client's positive thoughts and actions builds a healthy relationship. Genuine affirmations are used to strengthen the counselor–client connection.
5. *Rolling with resistance:* Acknowledging resistance often arising as a result of the counselor's style and not personal attributes of the client is crucial. Instead of confrontation, the counselor reframes the problem positively. For instance, "You don't want to upset your parents with personal problems, so you drink. Yet, they are disturbed by your drinking".
6. *Summarizing:* At intervals or session end, summarizing enhances clarity by reviewing narratives and exchanges. This helps consolidate information and highlights key points in the motivational interview process.

Step 2: Strengthening Commitment to Change

1. *Recognizing readiness to change:* In this determination stage, the counselor identifies signs of readiness in the client's behavior—settled demeanor, fewer questions, and self-motivational statements indicating a desire for change.
2. *Discussing a plan:* Transitioning from reasons to change, the counselor delves into action plans adjusted to the client's convenience. This stage involves collaboratively shaping a pathway for change.
3. *Communicating free choice:* Empowering the client, the counselor emphasizes the freedom to implement the change in their preferred way, giving a sense of responsibility. For instance, "It's entirely up to you how and when to go about this plan".
4. *Consequences of action and inaction:* To enhance awareness, a written list reflects the client's fears, expectations, and the pros

TABLE 3: A change worksheet.	
The changes I want to make are	
The most important reasons to make these changes are	
The specific steps I plan in making the change are	
Some people who can support me are	
They can help me by	
I will know how my plan is working when	
Things that could interfere with my plan (barriers) and possible solutions are	

and cons of behavior change. This tangible representation aids in comprehending the potential outcomes.

5. *Sharing a worksheet on planning change:* A structured approach is introduced through a planning worksheet **(Table 3)**, guiding the client in organizing thoughts and strategies for effective change in implementation.
6. *Providing relevant information:* Using an "Ask Share Ask" strategy, the counselor seeks permission, assesses the client's existing knowledge, and shares information accordingly. This respectful exchange ensures the client's engagement and comprehension.
7. *Supporting continued change:* Encouragement and support become essential in helping the client sustain the initiated change. Strategies involve affirmation, goal-focused discussions, and respect for the client's values. This ongoing support reinforces commitment and aids in the client's journey toward sustained positive change.

STRENGTHS OF MOTIVATIONAL INTERVIEWING

- Client-centric, gentle approach, widely accepted by individuals struggling with behavioral change
- Effective for patients with low motivation, hesitant to engage in structured therapies such as CBT

- Less time-consuming; 4 MI sessions equivalent to 12 sessions of CBT in treating disordered drinking
- Versatile application across various health-related issues, rehabilitation, public health, dentistry, coaching, and academics
- Demonstrated effectiveness in substance abuse treatment (alcohol, tobacco, and illicit drugs) and behavioral addictions such as gambling
- Useful in promoting healthy lifestyle changes for physical disorders (e.g., diabetes) and improving treatment compliance for chronic conditions (e.g., asthma).

LIMITATIONS OF MOTIVATIONAL INTERVIEWING

- Requires well-trained counselors; assessment tools such as motivational interviewing treatment integrity (MITI) are used in some countries.
- Challenges in maintaining equity as practitioners are in an expert role.
- Limited effectiveness in addressing severe mental disorders such as severe depression and suicidality.
- Less likely to be useful for adolescents under 12 due to neurodevelopmental and executive functioning prerequisites.

Relevance in adolescent office practice: MI is a teen-friendly intervention, respecting adolescent autonomy without being directive. It does not burden them with skill sets or assignments. MI enhances clinicians' communication and relationship-building skills, promoting patient compliance. For doctors, mastering MI techniques is rewarding, ensuring ongoing patient engagement and satisfaction in healthcare practice.

Motivational interviewing proves invaluable in counseling adolescents, creating rewarding and enjoyable interactions. By eliciting opinions and avoiding lectures, it taps into the resourcefulness of adolescents. MI empowers pediatricians to nurture autonomy, inculcate vital life skills, and encourage healthy choices without being preachy. Crucially, it builds a robust alliance, effectively tackling issues such as substance use. This ensures continued engagement with the healthcare system, preventing downstream complications and addressing problems at their root.

CONCLUSION

Motivational interviewing is a counselling approach based on humanitarian theories. It is employed in situations like substance abuse, weight reduction etc., wherein a behavioral change is aimed at. It works on the premise that the client is the best person to know himself and care for himself. The counsellor acts merely as a facilitator to bring about the desired change. He uses four spirits of MI, (collaboration, acceptance, compassion and evocation) to gently bring out the discrepancies in the client's values, goals and his current conduct. The motivation for change is thus just uncovered and the client is empowered to look after himself. The core principles, the skills that are employed during the sessions (the 'OARS') and the stepwise systematic methodology are the pillars of MI. With its client centric practical and flexible approach, it becomes a very suitable and acceptable form of talk therapy for adolescents and young adults.

SUGGESTED READING

1. Ghate S, Ghosh S. Motivational Interviewing Book. Adolescent Friendly Pediatric Practice. New Delhi: Jaypee Brothers Medical Publishers; 2023.
2. Hettema J, Steele J, Miller WR. Motivational interviewing. Annu Rev Clin Psychol. 2005;1:91-111.
3. Lundahl BW, Kunz C, Brownell C, Tollefson D, Burke BL. A meta-analysis of motivational interviewing: twenty-five years of empirical studies. Res Soc Work Pract. 2010;20:137-60.
4. Miller WR, Rollnick S. Motivational Interviewing: Preparing People for Change, 2nd edition. New York: Guilford Press; 2002.
5. Naar-King S, Suarez M. Motivational Interviewing with Adolescents and Young Adults. New York: Guilford Press; 2011.
6. Naar-King S. Motivational interviewing in adolescent treatment. Can J Psychiatry. 2011;56(11):651-7.
7. Prochaska J, Norcross J, Saul S. (2020). American Psychologist Generating Psychotherapy Breakthroughs: Transtheoretical

Strategies From Population Health Psychology. [online] Available from https://www.researchgate.net/publication/344862542_American_Psychologist_Generating_Psychotherapy_Breakthroughs_Transtheoretical_Strategies_From_Population_H [Last accessed September, 2024].

8. Resnicow K, McMaster F. Motivational interviewing: moving from why to how with autonomy support. Int J Behav Nutr Phys Act. 2012;9:19.
9. Rollnick, Miller WR, Butler CC. Motivational Interviewing in Health Care: Helping Patients Change Behavior. New York: Guilford Press; 2008.

16 CHAPTER

Counseling for Healthy Media Use

Shweta Sunil, Manoj Kumar Sharma, Narendra Nath Samantaray

INTRODUCTION

In today's digital age, where adolescents are immersed in a world of constant connectivity, the role of healthcare professionals extends beyond physical health to encompass the critical realm of healthy media use. Research underscores the vital role of counseling and parental involvement in shaping positive media habits among adolescents. Healthy media, particularly digital media, is essential for adolescents' well-being and academic success. Healthcare professionals play a crucial role in promoting healthy media use, balancing benefits and risks, and addressing unhealthy habits to ensure adolescents and their families adopt a healthy media use plan. In the following text, we introduce the structure and procedural details of counseling for healthcare professionals, with a focus on promoting healthy media use.

The foundational essence of counseling resides in the establishment of a professional helping relationship aimed at fostering the development of more proficient and adaptive behavior in clients. The following delineates the objectives of counseling across its developmental stages:

- *Relationship development:* In this initial stage, encompassing the inaugural encounter between the client and counselor, emphasis is placed on rapport building, information acquisition, goal delineation, and communication pertaining to counseling parameters. Within the context of counseling, this stage allows for the assessment of information related to an adolescent's media habits and exposure to diverse forms of media. Specific objectives involve the identification and establishment of concerns related to media use, such as excessive screen time, inappropriate content, or online safety.

- *Extended exploration:* Building upon the previous stage, this phase involves a more profound examination of personal, occupational, emotional, and cognitive dynamics in connection with the perceived benefits and impacts of media use on children.
- *Problem resolution:* Informed by preceding stages, this active phase entails the counselor's facilitation of change, wherein the client engages in re-evaluation, experimentation with new behaviors, and abandonment of those incongruent with established goals. In the pediatrician's role, evidence-based information on the impact of media on child development is shared, along with discussions on recommended strategies, such as adherence to screen time limits, the significance of coviewing or coengagement, and risk mitigation strategies addressing potential concerns such as exposure to inappropriate content, cyberbullying, and privacy issues. Tailored recommendations are contingent upon the child's age, interests, and family dynamics.
- *Termination and follow-up:* The concluding stage is collaboratively determined, with established methods for follow-up. The pediatrician may schedule subsequent appointments to assess progress and address emerging concerns, providing ongoing support and resources for parents (and also children) to navigate evolving digital trends.

CORE CONDITIONS OF COUNSELING RELATIONSHIPS

In order for counseling to succeed, a number of prerequisites must be met to maximize the beneficial effects of this helping connection. The following terms are typically used to describe these conditions: Empathic understanding, respect and positive regard, genuineness and congruence, warmth, and immediacy.

- *Empathic understanding:* Empathy involves an ability to understand clients' thoughts, feelings, and experiences from their perspective and communicate that understanding. It helps to connect with clients on an emotional level, build rapport, and gain insight into clients' concerns. The counselor strives to create an environment where the client perceives an accurate reflection of their thoughts and emotions.

- *Positive regards:* Respect and positive regard are the basic building blocks of the present counseling approach influenced by the seminal works of Rogers. It is characterized by a belief in the inherent worth and potential of each client, coupled with the ability to convey this belief to the client. Once conveyed, this idea gives clients encouragement regarding their intrinsic capacity to assume accountability for their own development, transformation, setting of goals, making decisions, and eventual problem-solving. Positive regard can boost a client's self-esteem and confidence in their ability to form effective relationships. A therapist's positive esteem can also encourage clients to participate in therapy, including tough self-disclosures and building resilience.
- *Genuineness and congruence:* In 1957, Carl Rogers viewed that for therapy to work, the person and therapist need to be in touch and understand each other. The therapist also needs to be genuine and have positive feelings toward the person. Rogers said that therapists should openly share their feelings without hiding behind a professional role. Being genuine, according to Rogers, means the therapist is aware of their own feelings and freely expresses them in therapy. This openness is important for building a real connection. In simpler terms, if a therapist is authentic and shares their feelings, it helps the therapy to be more effective. Hence, therapist congruence requires self-awareness, acceptance, and readiness to interact and communicate perceptions appropriately.
- *Warmth and immediacy:* Warmth in counseling is the genuine expression of care and concern for clients, indicating acceptance, a desire for their well-being, and sincere interest in finding solutions to their problems. Immediacy involves addressing present factors within the therapeutic relationship. This includes handling emotions such as anger or frustration as they arise. Managing these issues within the therapeutic relationship allows participants to gain insights into their behavioral patterns and

apply this understanding to relationships outside the counseling context, fostering personal growth.

SKILLS OF COUNSELOR

Active Listening

Active listening is a crucial skill in effective communication, particularly in counseling, encompassing both verbal and nonverbal elements to enhance communication and relationship building by demonstrating attentiveness, empathy, and understanding across various contexts. It goes beyond merely hearing words; it involves grasping the speaker's underlying emotions and intentions. Nonverbal cues such as eye contact, nodding, and appropriate facial expressions indicate engagement and attentiveness. Paraphrasing and summarizing the speaker's words confirm understanding and express empathy. Active listening also involves posing open-ended questions to encourage speakers to elaborate on their thoughts and emotions. This not only demonstrates interest in the speaker's perspective but also facilitates a deeper exploration of the subject.

It also involves using minimal encouragers. Minimal encouragers can be nonverbal cues that show that the counselor is paying attention to what is being stated, as well as spoken ones. A smile, a raised eyebrow, or a head nod are a few examples of nonverbal encouragers. Verbal minimal encouragers can be expressed with phrases such as "mmmm", "okay", "aha", "right", "I see", "oh?", "sure", "tell me more", "please continue", "really", and "yes". They can assist in providing counselor with more information and are helpful in encouraging the customer to speak further.

In counseling, active listening positively impacts client outcomes. Therapists employing active listening behaviors, including reflecting feelings and summarizing content, contribute to stronger empathy, therapeutic alliance, and increased client satisfaction.

Paraphrasing

Paraphrasing may be the most crucial information the client has just shared and reflecting them back is a useful technique for effectively explaining the material covered in an interview. The counselor literally replicates or reflects back to the clients what they have heard to apply this skill. Rather than verbatim repeating the client's remarks, the counselor uses his own words to reiterate the facts. Effective paraphrasing not only aids in verifying your comprehension of the communicated content but also assists the clients in elucidating their thoughts.

Following are usual steps of paraphrasing:

1. Use a sentence stem or opener to indicate that you will be providing feedback on what the client has been saying ("You appear to be saying...")
2. List the key points raised by the client (It seems you are frustrated with your son's use of mobile in the early morning...)
3. Verify if the client was accurately heard ("Am I right or something else...").

Reflection

This technique entails the counselor reflecting the client's core emotions while also verbalizing the sentiment expressed by the client. Feelings such as anger, depression, frustration, miserableness, tension, or franticness can be summed up in a single word, unlike thoughts, which frequently require a more detailed explanation. Reflecting on sentiments also demonstrates to the clients how well the counselor understands their experiences. Following are the components of reflection:

- Beginning of a sentence ("you seem to be..."; or "it seems you are... frustrated with your son's use of mobile in the early morning...)
- The use of emotive language (calm, sad, etc., such as, "it seems you are frustrated with your son's use of mobile in the early morning").
- Utilizing the present tense whenever feasible yields greater impact
- A query about correctness ("Am I right or something else...").

CONCLUSION

The cooperation of families and children is essential to the effective execution and maintenance of the advice given through counseling for appropriate media consumption. The families can adopt and modify the Family Media Use Plan as a flexible tool to help their adolescent children develop healthy media habits. Families are encouraged to actively engage in the creation of customized tactics that are suited to their child's age, interests, and family dynamics as the counseling process progresses. Scheduled follow-ups provide continued support and progress monitoring, extending the interaction that healthcare professionals and families build during counseling sessions outside the professional setting.

It is crucial to understand that certain circumstances could call for more knowledge, and doctors are prepared to refer patients to mental health specialists as needed. This cooperative strategy guarantees that families obtain all-encompassing assistance in managing potential mental health challenges as well as media-related issues. Families can effectively navigate the challenges of the digital age by promoting not only the well-being of adolescents but also the harmonious integration of media into their lives. This can be achieved through fostering open communication, putting recommended strategies into practice, and staying aware of how the digital landscape is changing. The implementation of suggested tactics, frequent check-ins, and a proactive approach to obtaining additional support when necessary all contribute to the long-term success of a healthy media use plan, especially as families strive to continue the counseling practice.

SUGGESTED READING

1. Beck K, Kulzer J. Teaching counseling microskills to audiology students: recommendations from professional counseling educators. Semin Hear. 2018;39(1):91-106.
2. Capuzzi D, Stauffer MD, Gross DR. The helping relationship: From core dimensions to brief and integrative possibilities. In: Capuzzi D, Stauffer MD (Eds). Counseling and Psychotherapy: Theories and Interventions. Alexandria: American Counseling Association; 2016. pp. 53-60.
3. Handel S. Listening as introduction to the perception of auditory events. Ear Hearing. 1990;11(3):243-7.
4. Rogers CR. The necessary and sufficient conditions of therapeutic personality change. J Consult Psychol. 1957;21(2):95-103.

17 CHAPTER

Trauma-informed Care

Sukanya Ray

INTRODUCTION

Trauma, literally meaning "wound", refers to the impact of critical events, *not the event itself.* The experience is characterized by a sense of helplessness and has a lasting impact on how one thinks, feels, and behaves. This chapter discusses different types of traumatic events and their effects, basic skills required for trauma-informed care (TIC), and stabilization techniques as a primary response by counselors to an adolescent with a traumatic experience.

Traumatic impact may be caused by *Big T, small t,* or *omission events.* Big T events are those that are prominent, discrete events that have a clear beginning and end such as accidents, physical assault, sexual assault, and bullying. Small t events are those that happen on an everyday basis for the individual such as arguments, fights, critical comments, and conflicts that are mostly invalidated and accepted by most people as "normal reality". Yet, these small t's cumulatively can have a lasting impact far greater than Big T's. Omission trauma refers to the events that were supposed to have happened in the course of a normal development but did not. These include neglect, invalidation of emotions, or absence of a nurturing attachment figure.

So, the concept of trauma is wider than the event-based criteria that exist for post-traumatic stress disorder (PTSD) as defined in the Diagnostic and Statistical Manual (DSM)-5. Complex PTSD (cPTSD), introduced by the International Classification of Diseases (ICD)-11, is an extension of the diagnostic category of PTSD and includes *disorders of self* (*DOS*) in addition to PTSD symptoms. These DOS symptoms signify persistent difficulties in understanding one's own self and in maintaining relationships. Complex trauma, introduced by Judith Herman, is a complex, multilayered presentation of the impact of various traumatic experiences—ranging from Big T's to small t's. It involves hidden wounds due to difficult relationships in childhood, adolescence, and early adulthood. It needs to be managed by experts trained in the areas of dissociation and trauma-focused approach.

The traumatic response is a neurobiological response. When an individual recalls a traumatic impact, or is triggered, the hypothalamic-pituitary-adrenal axis is activated, leading to a reactivation of the original traumatic response. This could manifest in the form of the defense cascade: Freeze → flight → fight → fright → flag → faint.

Daniel Siegel posited the model of the window of tolerance (WoT), which is useful in applying the understanding of Stephen Porges' polyvagal theory, in the context of counseling and psychotherapy. The polyvagal theory offers insights into how the vagus nerve performs regulatory functions in response to danger and safety cues detected by the nervous system. The WoT model proposes the existence of three zones based on vagal input **(Fig. 1)**:

1. *WoT:* This is the zone of optimal functioning, roughly corresponding to the ventral vagal system. This fosters social connection, relationships, and productivity. Minor triggers are managed by moving toward the edge of the WoT, either toward

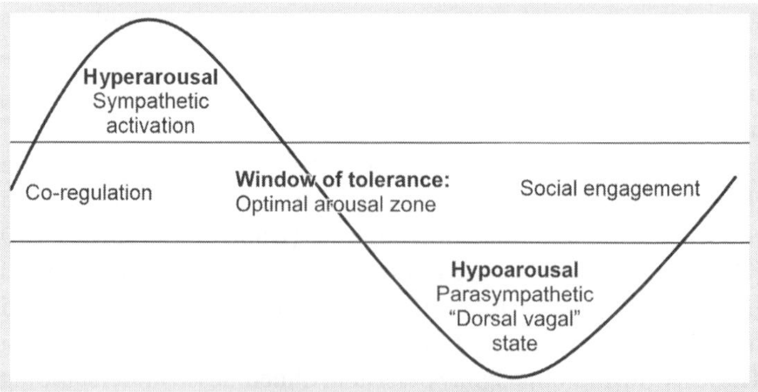

Fig. 1: Window of tolerance.

hyperarousal or hypoarousal. More intense triggers induce movement outside the window until the stressful impact is over.

2. *Hyperarousal:* This is the zone of mobilization or action—corresponding to the sympathetic system. Fight/flight/fawn/fend responses are prominent here—the emotions in this zone are activating in nature, pushing the individual to act on the traumatic stress, e.g., anger, anxiety, fear, and frustration.
3. *Hypoarousal:* This is the zone of immobilization or shutdown—corresponding to the dorsal vagal system. This can range from low activation states such as sadness/inattention/disorientation or zoning out/light dissociative states as well as flaccidity and faint responses. This also corresponds to feeling low energy and the inability to move or feeling "stuck".

States of hyperarousal and hypoarousal are natural adaptive states in response to stressors in the environment. When the danger/threat subsides, a return to optimal functioning or the WoT is natural and warranted. Traumatic experiences may interrupt this agile movement across zones and their recall may lead to a hyperarousal or hypoarousal and may also interrupt the "return" to WoT. Thus, people may experience feeling "stuck" in these hypo- or hyperemotions and may need a trauma-informed counseling approach to come back to their WoT.

TRAUMA-INFORMED APPROACH

Trauma-informed care is a transformational approach with its roots in the movement started by health personnel in the 1990s in the United States. TIC represents a significant shift from "what's wrong with you?" to a sensitive inquiry about "what happened to you?" TIC rests on the premise of *Primum non-nocere* or First Do No Harm. Being trauma-informed is not the same as being trauma-focused **(Table 1)**. First responders who may not be mental health professionals need information, learn trauma-informed handling, and make appropriate referrals to trauma-focused clinicians, as may be required. To be trauma-informed, counselors need to be informed of the following:

- Most counselees have been subjected to some form of trauma, e.g., violence, victimization, and/or invalidation in their present lives.

TABLE 1: Difference between trauma-informed and trauma-focused approaches.

Trauma-informed	*Trauma-focused*
Prevents retraumatization but does not engage in deep healing of trauma, does not involve "memory processing"	Prevents retraumatization and works toward healing the trauma, involves "memory processing"
Does not engage in addressing relational difficulties	Works toward healing core attachment wounds as the genesis of relational difficulties
Time-limited approach	Time-intensive approach
Resource-sensitive approach	Resource-intensive approach
Does not address core issues such as dissociation in complex trauma	Addresses and treats dissociation in complex trauma

- TIC is characterized by the values of safety, trustworthiness, choice, collaboration, and empowerment.

Inquisitiveness regarding events (*what happened*) and checklists of traumatic incidents may not be appropriate tools to approach an individual where traumatic impact is suspected. It is also impossible to assess the impact of trauma in the first interview with the client. It is important to *prevent retraumatization* during clinical interactions. Retraumatization essentially means activation of the trauma memory trace and resurgence of symptoms that could be linked to the traumatic impact. To prevent retraumatization, a sensitive and compassionate counseling style is essential. This style of counseling is characterized by the following:

- Active listening and following the underlying emotion. It is important to look for nonverbal signs of hyper- or hypoarousal—observe their tone/prosody/speed of speech and shifts in body language, posture, gestures, discomfort, tearing up, change in eye contact, any excitatory/inhibitory reflex, shrinking, or withdrawal. Each of these minute changes is telling signs and provides critical cues to prevent retraumatization.
- Validation of their present emotions and a safe space to facilitate trust-building, e.g., "your feelings of sadness and grief are

natural—anyone in your place would have had the same feelings". or "It makes sense to me that you are still scared/anxious/sad about this". Due to their history of having difficult relationships, individuals may need repeated use of empathy and collaboration to be able to build trust and safety.

- Being sensitive to trauma narratives. There is often a need in the adolescent to *feel seen* and share the pain they have endured. However, merely hearing the client's story does more harm than good. A sensitive clinician learns to be aware of potential retraumatization and avoids detailed sharing. Sometimes, this may involve the clinician taking on the role of a parent talking "tough love" exemplified in such statements as "I know you want me to hear you out and that is important too. Yet it's far more important for me to not get your mind into the whirlpool of that painful experience and memories—that could cause you more damage. I can suggest an alternate approach that has been found to be useful in dealing with the difficulties you are holding..." Or "Let's ensure you have what it takes to talk about the pain—sometimes we need resources to hold us when we narrate out our pain. These are called resourcing/stabilization skills and will prevent further pain for you".
- Avoid detailed questioning of the time of the impact—asking details about what happened, how they felt, what they saw, what they did, or what they thought—all of which may be retraumatizing. While general questions about the age and a general sense of danger can be used, details are to be avoided to avoid bringing up the traumatic memory. Instead, questions that can assess the current impact can be asked: "When you think/talk about it *now*, as of date, what are you left thinking/feeling/experiencing about it?"
- Psychoeducation regarding the trauma-informed approach, the neurobiological response WoT, and helping them to return to their optimal state or WoT using stabilization techniques is required.
- Avoid giving false hopes or expert advice. Instead provide information, counseling, and whenever required referral to a trauma-focused clinician.

- Avoid the word "trauma" to avoid stigmatization and use words such as difficulty/pain using the client's own words that are culturally appropriate.
- Avoid the use of words such as "willpower", "choice", "determination", or "strength"—these words do not empower individuals and may instead contribute to their feeling of helplessness.

STABILIZATION

Stabilization techniques can be essentially grouped into two categories: *Downregulating* techniques that help in *bringing down* the neural activation from the hyperarousal state to the WoT and *upregulating* techniques that help in *bringing up* the neural activation from the hypoarousal state to the WoT. Downregulation techniques to bring down sympathetic activation may involve working with the body, such as breathing, sighing, yawning, light stroking on the deltoid muscles, or using external resources such as relaxation scripts (progressive muscular relaxation, guided imagery, cued relaxation, etc.), activating the mammalian dive reflex by dipping or washing the face with cold water, etc.

Upregulation techniques involve *grounding*, such as by orienting them to the time, surroundings, and familiar objects in the environment, inviting them to explore the environment with their olfactory and tactile senses. It could also involve the body directly—rubbing hands together, small movements that facilitate lengthening of the spine, small movements of the eye muscles and/or neck, or placing the feet firmly on the ground.

CONCLUSION

Trauma is not in the event but what has stayed on from the experience into the present. TIC is a sensitive, collaborative approach that ensures safety, dignity, and agency of the counselee. It involves specific skills to prevent retraumatization and ensure stabilization. Return to the window of optimal arousal is the key to achieving stabilization. After providing the initial counseling, referral to a mental health professional with expertise in trauma-informed approach may be considered.

SUGGESTED READING

1. Corrigan FM, Fisher JJ, Nutt DJ. Autonomic dysregulation and the window of tolerance model of the effects of complex emotional trauma. J Psychopharmacol. 2011;25:17-25.
2. Fisher J. The work of stabilization in trauma treatment. Paper presented at The Trauma Center Lecture Series, 1999. [online] Available from https://www.complextrauma.uk/uploads/2/3/9/4/23949705/the_work_on_stabilization_in_trauma_work.pdf [Last accessed September, 2024].
3. Kezelman C, Stavropoulos P. Organizational Guidelines for Trauma-Informed Service Delivery. Sydney: Blue Knot Foundation; 2020.
4. MacLean PD. The Triune Brain in Evolution: Role in Paleocerebral Functions. New York: Springer; 1990.
5. Porges SW. Orienting in a defensive world: mammalian modifications of our evolutionary heritage. A polyvagal theory. Psychophysiology. 1995;32:301-18.
6. Porges SW. Polyvagal theory: a science of safety. Front Integr Neurosci. 2022;16:871227.
7. Schauer M, Elbert T. Dissociation following traumatic stress. J Psychol. 2010;218(2):109-27.
8. Siegel DJ. The Developing Mind: Toward a Neurobiology of Interpersonal Experience. New York; The Guilford Press; 1999.
9. Steffen PR, Hedges D, Matheson R. The brain is adaptive not triune: how the brain responds to threat, challenge and change. Front Psychiatry. 2022;13:802606.

18 CHAPTER

Scholastic Counseling

Mini K Paul, Mercy Sebastian

INTRODUCTION

Learning is a lifelong process, the basis of which is life experiences. Good academic performance requires basic intelligence, an environment conducive to learning and appropriate learning techniques. There are different learning or understanding styles: (1) Visual learners—learn better by reading line by line and word by word, (2) auditory learners—learn better by reading aloud, and (3) experiential learners—learn better by experiencing or experimenting. An individual child may use all modalities of learning, but at the same time may have any of the three learning styles. In the school system, we do not differentiate the learning styles of individual children; hence, we need to provide all three modalities at the same time. The teacher needs to speak aloud, write notes on the board, and conduct simple experiments in the class or give life experiences in the community. Before counseling a child, we also need to understand whether the child has a predominant left or right brain function.

LEFT BRAIN FUNCTIONS

Use of right hands, indicates predominant functions of reasoning-sequencing, software, scientific skills, mathematics numbers, reading-spelling-writing language, listening-speaking language, and languages to convert ideas to spoken or written form.

RIGHT BRAIN FUNCTIONS

Use of left hand, indicates predominant functions of motors-machines, dance, music and its appreciation, acting-mimicking, fantasy, imagination, storytelling, designing, crafting, building, sports, games, using maps-piloting-navigating, perception-fixing names to faces, sculpture-art and its appreciation, painting-appreciation, cooking, homemaking, and leadership-management-life skills. Naturally, a person with predominant right brain functions is not likely to excel in academics but would show a flair for sports, games, arts, music, and literature.

IMPROVING MEMORY

Most children would complain of not being able to remember the class lessons. To counsel these children, we need to understand the functions of brain and the process of learning. At the time of birth, the neuronal connections in the brain are not too many but by 2 years, they become very dense, with a lot of experiences in the first 2 years of life. The neuronal connections form the pathway for information transfer, processing, and recall. The more you read, write, or experience, the denser would be the neuronal connections. This can be compared to your trying to find a house in a "city ward". If you have gone alone asking the way or if you have gone a few times to the same house, you cannot forget the way for a long time. But if somebody had been dropping you there in a vehicle, then you may not remember the way, even if you had gone there many times. The study process is also similar; you have to learn by yourself and repeat the same again and again; you will never forget it in the examination.

Tips for Improving Memory

- Make associations—mnemonics, mind maps
- Make key points—pocketbook, flash cards
- Graphic representations
- Connect related topic and read
- Combined study
- Teach someone else—mother using black/whiteboard.

SQ3R method can be used to improve textbook comprehension. SQ3R is an acronym that stands for survey, questions, read, recall, and review. First, all the key points and diagrams of a particular chapter are surveyed. Then each bold heading in the chapter is converted to a question. Answers are read and then written in the student's language. Then the student recalls the answer. In the end, the entire chapter is reviewed. Portions that are not mastered are reread.

SCHOLASTIC BACKWARDNESS

Scholastic achievement is what is close to the heart of any parent. Hence, the best opportunity or window of access to adolescent problems is through scholastic underachievement, focusing on the child with "red marks" in the progress card and digging out problems one by one. Teen club/adolescent club in the school is a viable strategy to focus on academic issues in the garb of extracurricular activities under the guidance of a teacher and with support of a professional counselor.

When children are required to engage in academic exercises that require attention, specific cognitive abilities and processes, and demonstrations of learning, a subset of these children are unable to perform due to some type of intellectual, emotional, behavioral, physical, or environmental deficit. Any combination of these factors can result in school failure. Children differ in their academic achievements. Academic achievement refers to the knowledge attained or skill developed in the school subjects usually assessed by test scores, or by marks assigned by teachers or by both. Underachievement or the inability to perform up to one's intelligence level may be due to various factors, which may include factors in the child and factors in the environment. Scholastic backwardness or poor academic performance in children may be due to various reasons.

Study Habits

We teach our children a whole lot of subjects but never bother to teach them how to study. Learning skill is an important factor in developing proper study habits. Much of individual success in life depends upon the care and confidence with which one acquires knowledge and upon one's ability to perform tasks. Learning depends largely upon intelligence and motivation, and motivation depends on the need a student must feel to learn.

Study habits or the way in which a student approaches his studies and the importance given to his/her studies can have great influence on academic achievement. Studies conducted by Nair MKC et al., on scholastic backwardness among adolescents of rural, urban, and residential high schools have shown that >50% (51–73%) of the students are not studying their daily lessons. Reasons given for postponing their daily studies are:

- Not getting enough time to complete daily studies
- Not bothered to study their daily lessons
- Spending more time on extracurricular activities
- Perceived headaches and other illnesses, etc.

Staying attentive in class or being free from other distractions is another important factor. It was also revealed that many students had problems regarding staying attentive in class. Major distractions or reasons reported by the students for lack of concentration while attending class were:

- Thinking about other things
- Not able to understand lessons
- Personal worries
- Boredoms.

Though these types of distractions are common at this age, their adverse effect on scholastic performance can be reduced by effective teacher–student interaction and by using better study habits.

Tips for Promoting Good Study Habits

- Time management—make a daily timetable by listing time spent in sleeping, grooming, meals, errands, school, television, meeting with friends, play, and hobbies. The remaining time can be planned for studies. Study time can be divided into time for doing homework, daily revision of lessons, and extra reading.
- Have a regular study pattern—read tomorrow's topic once today, read daily lessons, and revise.
- Better concentration—write down key points and repeat them many times.
- Reduce personal factors/distractions in studies—set targets and insist on meeting the targets.

- Promote ambition and motivation—internal (from within) and external (enabling environment).

Intelligence

Children differ in their intellectual ability, and intellectual ability is an important factor in determining the academic performance of a student. The term "intelligence" refers to an individual's ability to cope with its environment through learning and can be assessed by various standardized tests. There are many factors that influence the intellectual development of a person, including biological as well as environmental factors. It may be helpful to have an idea about the intellectual ability of the student before dealing with his/her scholastic problems.

Physical Health

The physical health of a child reflects on his/her overall growth and personality development. Chronic health problems can affect the learning and academic performance of a student. Prolonged malnutrition can be a cause for poor achievement, and iron deficiency anemia in infants can lead to developmental problems. A study conducted in the United States to investigate the relationship between iron deficiency and cognitive test scores among a nationally representative sample of 5,398 school-aged children and adolescents had shown that 3% were iron-deficient, the prevalence being the highest among adolescent girls (8.7%). Average mathematics scores were lower for children with iron deficiency with and without anemia, compared with children with normal iron status. By logistic regression, children with iron deficiency had greater than twice the risk of scoring below average in mathematics than did children with normal iron status. It is of utmost importance to note that this elevated risk was present even for iron-deficient children without anemia.

Frequent or prolonged illness causes absence from school, which may result in poor academic performance or failure. Some of the common symptoms/problems experienced by adolescents are headache, chest pain, abdominal pain, or dizziness that may be psychophysiological responses to stress, anxiety, depression, etc. To deal with these problems, in addition to a careful medical assessment, the evaluation must include a review of psychosocial functioning in the family, school, peer group, community, etc., using the HEEADSSS (Home, Education/employment, Eating, Activities, Drugs, Sexuality, Suicidal ideation, and Safety) framework (see Chapter 7). Appropriate management may include supportive counseling, instruction in relaxation techniques, and, if required, medication.

Family Environment

Parents and family environment play an important role in the academic performance of a student. Studies have shown that the parents' involvement and concern stimulate their children to do better at school. Some of the factors related to family that can influence the academic achievement of a student are:

- Emotional environment
- Physical environment
- Motivation
- Help in studies from parents, siblings, or others
- Education status of parents
- Chronic illness of family members, etc.

School Environment

Most activities of human beings are designed to make them more comfortable, happy, and peaceful in their relationship with the environment. This involves adjustment to external and internal conditions. Happiness at school is an essential prerequisite for academic achievement. Children of poor social background fail to achieve full potential in school. The quality and amount of home support play an important role in academic achievement. Poverty combined with a low self-image seems to damage students' achievement, motivation, and self-respect. The school is an institution, espousing middle-class values, and the teachers tend to appreciate more middle-class values of conformity and obedience. It is in this context that it has become almost mandatory to have counseling services provided at schools.

Specific Learning Disability

Specific learning disability (SLD) is characterized by significant delays in one or more areas of the learning process in a child of normal or above-normal intelligence. SLD may present as neurological disorders, behavioral disorders, and scholastic backwardness.

The American Academy of Child and Adolescent Psychiatry has opined that parents should be aware of the most frequent signals of learning disabilities when a child:

- Has difficulty in understanding and following instructions
- Has trouble in remembering what someone has just told him or her
- Fails to master reading, spelling, writing, and/or math skills, and thus, fails schoolwork
- Has difficulty in distinguishing right from left; difficulty in identifying words or a tendency to reverse letters, words, or numbers (e.g., confusing 25 with 52, "b" with "d", or "on" with "no")
- Lacks coordination in walking, sports, or simple activities such as holding a pencil or tying a shoelace
- Easily loses or misplaces homework, schoolbooks, or other items
- Cannot understand the concept of time; is confused by "yesterday", "today", and 'tomorrow".

Children with learning disabilities usually have a normal range of intelligence. They try very hard to follow instructions, concentrate, and "be good" at home and in school. However, despite this effort, he or she is not mastering school tasks and falls behind. It is believed that learning disabilities are caused by a difficulty with the nervous system that affects receiving, processing, or communicating information, which may also run in families. Some children with learning disabilities are also hyperactive; unable to sit still, easily distracted, and have a short attention span. Children with learning disabilities need special attention and treatment. If not detected and treated early, however, they can have a tragic "snowballing" effect. The child, trying very hard to learn, becomes more and more frustrated and develops emotional problems such as low self-esteem in the face of repeated failures. Some learning-disabled children misbehave in school because they would rather be seen as "bad" than "stupid" and each misbehavior needs correction by a professional counselor.

CONCLUSION

It may be noted that adolescents, parents, and teachers need to be counseled about the importance of ensuring age-appropriate sleep, nutrition, physical activity, sleep, study skills, healthy media use, stress management techniques, pursuing hobbies, annual wellness visits, completing age-appropriate vaccination, and a nurturing school and family environment. An individualized education plan (IEP) may be formulated for adolescents with SLD, intellectual disability, and attention-deficit/hyperactivity disorder (ADHD) by a remedial educator. After disability certification, these students can avail of special privileges by state and central boards in the form of extra time for completion of exams, subject exemption, use of a calculator, and scribe for exams. A few of them may opt to join the National Institute of Open Schooling (NIOS). Under the NIOS scheme, a wide array of academic and vocational subjects is offered and the students can complete their secondary education at their own pace with minimal stress.

SUGGESTED READING

1. Bukatko D, Daehler MW. Child Development: A Thematic Approach, 3rd edition. New York: Houghton Mifflin Company; 1998.
2. Galagali PM. Study skills. In: Choudhry J (Ed). Behavioral Problems in Children and Adolescents, 2nd edition. New Delhi: Jaypee Brothers Medical Publishers; 2024. pp. 249-64.
3. Galagali PM, Luiz N. School performance in adolescence. In: Pemde H, Ratna Kumari TL, Galagali PM, Velmurugan (Eds). Adolescent Friendly Pediatric Practice. New Delhi: Jaypee Brothers Medical Publishers; 2024. pp. 225-36.
4. Good CV (Ed). Dictionary of Education. New York: McGraw-Hill; 1973.
5. Nair MKC. CDC-UNICEF-ADOL Project Report. Trivandrum: Child Development Centre; 2001.
6. Nair MKC. Teenage morbidity in the community. In: Pejaver RK (Ed). Adolescent Care 2000 and beyond. Bengaluru: Prism Books Ltd; 2000. pp. 81-98.

19 CHAPTER

Guidance and Counseling in School Setting

Mini K Paul, Suresh Kumar G

INTRODUCTION

Guidance is assistance given to a person to make effective, individually satisfying, and socially acceptable choices. The adolescent has needs, so do the people around him/her, and both are complementary. Adjustment is the process of establishing a satisfactory psychological relationship between the individual and the environment. The ability to adjust is not innate and has to be developed.

PRINCIPLES OF GUIDANCE

Guidance is a slow, continuous, and ongoing process. The general direction is preventive in nature, helping individuals to develop insight. Guidance is an organized service that can also solve some of the minor problems, utilizing experiences of the individuals or others around them. If there is a desirable outcome, the same strategy may be used again later on, and if the outcome is undesirable, try to use a different strategy. Guidance can also be advising, which sometimes does have positive results. In a nutshell, guidance:

- Concentrates on the person rather than on the problem
- Tries to identify the abilities and limitations of the person
- Leads to self-development and self-direction
- Helps an individual make necessary adjustments
- Helps an individual achieve happiness and success.

NEED FOR GUIDANCE SERVICES

- To select educational courses or career and the desirability of each course, and to identify the suitable one

- To settle difference of opinion on choice of career between the parents and the adolescents
- To mediate between needs of rural children and educational environment in the towns/cities
- To bring a balance between educational environment and capabilities of the adolescent child
- To help young people (10–24 years) make adjustments, bring emotional stability, and avoid strained relations
- To guide adolescents cope with changing interests, attitudes, and perceptions
- To help adolescents facing problems related to early puberty and late puberty by trying to change attitude of parents and teachers
- To identify causes of misbehavior and to help parents and teachers solve problems amicably
- To help make effective decision by understanding and evaluating problems
- To help adolescents who are afraid of taking decisions, because of the impact of negative decisions taken in the past.

ROLE OF GUIDANCE WORKER

Guidance is an organized function that facilitates the personal development of an individual and seeks cooperation of others like teachers, parents, friends, relatives, and specifically the guidance worker, who should understand the problem first and then make teachers and parents understand the same. It is achieved through observation, i.e., information received by all the sense organs, and not by measurement with any instrument or tool. Guidance workers do not manipulate or change anything. They may take a structured or unstructured, formal or informal, and participatory or nonparticipatory approach. The steps in guidance are planning, observing, recording, analyzing, and concluding. If there is more than one observer, all have to be equally trained to make unbiased observations. However, the number of traits to be observed should be limited. In the home or school situation, the norms, values, belief systems, culture, love, and affection, all have to be observed carefully before analysis.

Objectives of Guidance and Counseling Services in Schools

Educational Guidance

- To monitor the academic progress of students studying in the institution
- To enable students to get an insight into their potential, strengths, and weaknesses for learning
- To assist students in getting information about further education and training
- To identify "weak students", diagnose their learning difficulties, and organize remedial measures
- To identify special learners such as the creative and gifted and cater to their needs and development.

Social and Psychological Guidance

- To identify students who have problems of adjustment and help them resolve the same
- To inculcate proper values, habits, attitudes, and temperament for studies and work
- To assist in developing interpersonal relationships among students
- To guide students in using leisure time profitably and usefully
- To assist students in maintaining sound mental health.

Vocational/Career Guidance

- To collect and disseminate information about job opportunities to students
- To assist students develop the ability to analyze occupational information and make appropriate occupational choice
- To provide information to students about self-employment opportunities.

Educational Guidance

Educational guidance is aimed at assisting students make decisions and solve problems pertaining to their educational progress and development. It would be appropriate to start giving assistance at the last year of their high school as some of the problems of college students have their origin at this stage. Decision regarding continuation of education and selection of course and college are made by the students in this stage. Some of the important data needed for educational guidance are as follows:

- *College records:* The official records kept for administrative purpose in the college contain facts about every student's background, academic history, health, and hobbies.
- *Informal teacher/parent report:* Apart from the formal reports, teachers can supply helpful guidance information through informal reports of their observations of pupil behavior during classroom hours. Parents can also give information regarding students' general tendencies, likes and dislikes, and strengths and weaknesses.
- *Student self-reports:* The perceptions of a student of his/her own self are important data for education guidance. Self-reported data can be obtained on almost all aspects of one's educational life.
- *Use of standardized tests:* A well-planned and administered program of guidance also requires objective data on every student. Objective data pertaining to an individual's abilities, interests, aptitudes, personality, and attitude are obtainable through the use of standardized tests of measurement.

Role of Parents and Teachers in Guiding Students

Parents and teachers play a key role in ensuring that their child or adolescent achieves school success. When parents, students, and staff work together, the student will achieve his/her academic goals. Some of the actions that parents and teachers can take to promote school success are given in the following text.

Academic Work

- Parents can discuss with the teachers their children's problems in studies.
- Discuss his/her general behavior pattern at school
- Parents and teachers can help students set clear expectations for studies and future.

- Teachers can help students to learn difficult subjects by providing opportunity for clarification of doubts and arranging peer tutoring.

Interpersonal Relations/Peer Interaction

- Parents and teachers can observe the nature of friendships of students.
- Encourage children to associate with positive role models.
- The schools can arrange teen clubs with participation of students, teachers, and parent representatives.
- As part of teen club activities, personality development/life skill training can be arranged for students.

Family Atmosphere

- Provide a healthy family atmosphere.
- Try to do something enjoyable with your child at least once a week and spend quality time with your child.
- Create an atmosphere at home where children are free to talk everything about themselves at least to one parent or a responsible elder person.

Parent–Teacher Relations

- Get acquainted with your child's teachers.
- Communicate with school staff when there is a concern with the school adjustment/studies.
- Ensure parents' participation in school activities.

Participation in Extracurricular Activities

- Encourage students to participate in school-related activities.
- Encourage students to talk about school, social activities, and their interests.
- Teachers can encourage shy students also to take part in group activities by allotting small responsibilities.

Moral Values

- Teach standards of right and wrong as is appropriate socially and culturally.

- Make students aware of their responsibilities, to themselves, family, and society.
- Support school discipline policies.

Healthy Habits

- Parents and teachers can talk to the students about tobacco, drugs, and alcohol and about their adverse effects.
- Monitor your child's preference of friends, choices of leisure time activity, TV programs, etc.
- Arrange talks/educational programs on good habits, health, and hygiene practices.

Health-related Aspects

- Provide age-appropriate knowledge on growth and nutrition aspects.
- School parent–teacher association or teen club can arrange periodic health checkup/immunization programs.
- Provide reproductive and sexual health education.
- Service of a school counselor is a must to make a difference in dealing with common issues/problems seen in the school setting.

Guidance Tips for Handling Common Behavioral Concerns of Students School Refusal

Some students show reluctance to attend school for various reasons with varying intensity levels. In some cases, they need expert psychological intervention to solve the problem. Possible causes include enmeshed or overly protective parents, traumatic events, neglectful or inconsistent environment, and lax discipline.

Students with this problem may show:

- Reluctance to attend school because of the desire to stay at home
- Emotional distress when thinking about school
- Somatic complaints associated with attending school or anticipation of school
- Excessive clinging to/overdependence on parents
- Repeatedly asking the necessity for attending school

- Fear that something bad will happen at home if he/she goes to school.

How to Help

- Parents must encourage (not forcefully/compelling) the student to go to school every day.
- Parents and teachers can discuss with the child about his/her feelings and worries associated with attending school.
- Encourage good/healthy friendship in class and school.
- Teachers can give the child an opportunity to assist him/her in setting special projects/activities that he/she will enjoy.
- Help them set realistic achievable ambition.
- Teachers can support the student to develop secure feeling at school.
- If none of the above works, counseling by a qualified counselor/ clinical psychologist and, in a few cases, medication may be indicated.

Academic Underachievement

Academic underachievement is a condition in which the student is not able to perform up to his/her abilities in academic performance, due to various reasons. Possible causes include poor study habits, not following a systematic study pattern, low intellectual capacity, depression or low self-esteem, learning disability, health-related issues (physical and mental), and adjustment problems at school. Students with academic underachievement may show:

- Lack of interest in studies
- Lack of concentration in studies—too many distractions
- Do not complete school or homework assignments on time
- Heightened anxiety that interferes with the student's performance during tests
- No systematic study habits
- Repeated failure in one or more subjects
- Academic performance is below the student's apparent intelligence level.

How to Help

- Ensure that the student is following a systematic study pattern—help develop effective study skills and monitor academic progress.
- Parents should ensure to maintain regular (at least monthly) communication with teachers to help the student remain organized and keep up with assignments.
- Provide necessary help and support in studying weak subjects.
- Set short- and long-term goals.
- Discuss the student's negative attitude toward studies. Focus on changing that attitude.
- Teach test-taking skills—practice model tests frequently.
- Direct student to use planners to record school assignments and daily study pattern and plan ahead for long-term projects.
- Encourage parents to give compliments and positive reinforcements for the student's efforts and academic success.
- If required, refer the student for medical examination.
- If none of the above works, counseling by a qualified counselor/clinical psychologist and, in a few cases, medication may be indicated.

Low Self-esteem

Many studies have shown that self-esteem and academic achievement are positively correlated. Students with low self-esteem may have various adjustment problems also. Generally, students with low self-esteem:

- Cannot identify positive traits or personal talents
- Refuse to take positive risks associated with new experiences
- Lack self-confidence
- Excessively seek to please or receive attention
- Act out in negative, attention-seeking ways
- Avoid social contact with adults and peers

Possible causes include being a perfectionist (resulting in a feeling of inadequacy and frustration when the goals are not reached), genetic (low self-esteem might run in the family), anger turned inward (will not directly express anger), rarely experienced success (feels worthless because of many failures), overprotected (have not learned how to cope), does not feel respected and feel neglected (results in feeling of worthlessness), and an autocratic or punishing environment (feels helpless and believes that the world is a bad place).

How to Help

- Provide warmth, empathy, and acceptance; encourage expression of feelings at home and at school.
- Use puppets, art, or role-plays to play out scenes such as starting conversations, taking positive risks, expressing feelings, or asking for something that she/he needs.
- Focus on positives; model optimism.
- Foster self-understanding, competency, and independence.
- Find activities in which the individual will experience constructive endeavors and enjoyable activities.
- Identify instances in which self-esteem has been damaged and help the individual think about other possible ways to overcome that situation.
- Practice accepting and acknowledging compliments.
- Ask the student to write one positive thing about himself/herself daily. Have him/her realize that he/she has over 100 things about which to be proud of.
- If none of the above works, counseling by a qualified counselor/clinical psychologist and, in a few cases, medication may be indicated.

Anxiety

Anxiety is experienced by everyone. While minimum anxiety is constructive, intense anxiety can be crippling. Overanxiety due to various reasons is a major cause of poor academic performance in many students. Possible causes include traumatic experience in life; projected anger (e.g., if physically abused); physiological (central nervous system highly reactive); perfectionist (standards too high); inconsistent, neglectful, or confusing environment; and personality problems. Students with excessive anxiety may have:

- A specific fear that significantly interferes with the student's daily life
- Rapid heartbeat, shortness of breath, dizziness, nausea, or digestion problems (autonomic symptoms)
- Concentration difficulties, trouble sleeping, and irritability

How to Help

- Identify specific worries, fears, and anxieties.
- Use behavioral techniques to face fears. If a student is fearful of going outside (agoraphobic), ask him/her to draw a picture of going outside. Then have him/her imagine going outside. Ask him/her to take one step outside. Increase the steps and amount of time outside, until he/she is not fearful of going outside. Do not rush this process. It may take weeks or longer.
- Be firm, encouraging, and compassionate.
- Promote security; provide a consistent and caring environment.
- Explore distorted cognitive messages that mediate the anxiety response.
- Encourage the expression of feelings.
- Use art, play, or role-plays to practice strategies of handling anxiety and fears.
- Encourage the student to participate in extracurricular activities that involve exercise and healthy friendships.
- Provide a consistent, nurturing, and dependable environment.
- Teach relaxation and cognitive diversion.
- If none of the above works, counseling by a qualified counselor/ clinical psychologist and, in a few cases, medication may be indicated.

Anger

Adolescents may, sometimes, show overt expression of anger more than others. When it comes to a stage where they are not able to control, it may result in adjustment/behavioral problems and low achievement levels. Intervention is required at this stage to help them. Possible causes include emotions building up and then blowing off; being exposed to a frustrating or hostile environment;

learned behavior (got desired results in the past from throwing a tantrum); underlying feelings of depression, anxiety, or insecurity; and part of personality problem. These adolescents may express:

- Anger outbursts that are out of proportion to the precipitating events
- Strained interpersonal relationships with family members and peers due to aggressiveness and anger
- Verbal threats to siblings, peers, or adult authority figures
- Frequent fighting or arguing
- Pattern of destroying property or throwing objects

How to Help

- Teach how to diffuse anger early and how to appropriately express minor irritations immediately.
- Use therapeutic anger games to assist the student in becoming more verbal about feelings.
- Examine the core conflicts that are contributing to the anger problems.
- Assist the parents in establishing rules and consequences for the student's angry outbursts.
- Use art, play, or role-plays to practice strategies to handle anger.
- Encourage participation in extracurricular activities that provide a physical outlet.
- Use the empty chair technique to express anger about past or current people that make the student angry.
- Assist students to identify successful strategies they have used in the past to control their temper.
- Place students in an anger counseling group to improve anger control and interpersonal skills.
- If none of the above works, counseling by a qualified counselor/clinical psychologist and, in a few cases, medication may be indicated.

Shyness

Shyness is a problem faced by many children, especially adolescents. Shy children may not achieve success in life according to their potentials. Shyness interferes with learning, developing self-esteem, socialization, and psychological adjustment. Possible causes include often being criticized or teased; overprotected, neglectful, or disinterested parents; and personality problems. Shy children may show:

- Limited eye contact, refusal to respond to others, and isolation in social situations
- Few close friendships outside the immediate family members
- Hypersensitivity to criticism or perceived signs of rejection
- Excessive need for reassurance
- Reluctance to engage in new activities
- Negative self-image
- *Physiological distress in social settings:* Sweating, trembling, increased heart rate.

How to Help

- Encourage expression of feelings.
- Actively build a level of trust with the student through eye contact, empathy, and listening.
- Create an environment that enhances self-esteem and social interactions at school and at home.
- Teach social skills and make opportunity to practice them.
- Use art, play, or role-plays to express feelings and practice social interactions.
- Find activities where am individual will experience constructive endeavors and enjoyable activities.
- Identify instances where self-esteem has been damaged.
- Ask the student to write one positive thing about himself/herself daily. Have him/her realize that he/she has more than 100 things about which to be proud of.
- Help him/her to set goals and monitor progress.
- If required, refer for a speech/language evaluation to rule out impairment that may lead to shyness.
- If none of the above works, counseling by a qualified counselor/ clinical psychologist and, in a few cases, medication may be indicated.

VOCATIONAL DEVELOPMENT

The three stages of vocational development in terms of occupational decision-making are as follows:

1. Fantasy choice stage
2. Tentative choice stage
3. Realistic choice stage.

The *fantasy choice stage* is between 6 and 11 years of age. The children at this stage exercise their occupational choices more on fantasy. They verbally express their ideas as fantasies of what they like to do when they grow up. They primarily think of an activity which will give them pleasure.

The *tentative choice* stage ranges from 12 to 16 years. At this stage, the child brings about changes in his/her vocational choice.

The *realistic choice* stage starts around the age of 17 years which may be considered as late adolescence and continues through early adulthood. At this stage, one makes efforts to explore the world around with a view to make a wiser and more stable choice. One becomes more and more aware of one's likes and dislikes and also the societal forces and obligations which eventually crystallize one's choice. The availability of job and economic circumstances in which the individual is placed are also important factors influencing one's career.

VOCATIONAL/CAREER GUIDANCE

Career planning and occupational choice are of primary importance in a student's life for a better future. Sometimes, occupations are selected arbitrarily and accidentally, leading to many frustrations in future life. In every decision of occupational choice, the individual himself/herself and many others are involved, the parents, teachers, friends, etc. Sometimes the parents force the individual in pursuing a career, although it may not conform to his/her interest or aptitude.

How Occupational Choices are Made

The first and most generally accepted theory of occupational choice says that the individual makes decision about career choice "accidentally"—something beyond his/her control. The accident theory stresses the importance of external factors in the choice process.

How to Make the Choice of a Career

The proper selection of a career would require the student to have:

- A complete understanding of himself/herself as much as possible
- A complete knowledge of the occupation as much as possible
- An ability to match what he/she possesses and what is required.

In order to have a complete analysis of them, students should make an honest subanalysis. They should obtain an objective analysis of themselves from teachers and parents on what they have observed. If possible, consult an expert such as a guidance worker to get a scientific analysis, through the administration of appropriate tests.

A complete knowledge of an occupation would depend on the person's awareness about the occupational description and requirements. One ought to know about the nature of work one is expected to do in the occupation and the duties and responsibilities involved in it. Sometimes, an occupation requires special abilities and one should know whether there is any such thing involved in the occupation under consideration. Some occupations require special educational qualifications.

- A knowledge about essential and desirable qualification
- Time of notification/application
- How to apply
- About interview/entrance test
- Restrictions, if any, such as marital status, age, sex, and reservations
- Working conditions: Regular hours of work, leave facilities, salary and perks, promotional avenues, vacation, housing, etc.

Common Mistakes in Career Choice

An Arbitrary Decision

The college/university education necessitates a student to prepare and opt for vocation. The commitment begins when the student selects a particular stream and course for study and puts into action when he/she joins an occupation. Most of the students make a crucial decision under considerable stress and confusion. The result is more of an arbitrary selection than a systematically planned one.

Choosing an Occupation without Appropriate Abilities and Personality Makeup

Every occupation requires certain abilities and personality characteristics. Success in the occupation to a large extent depends on whether the aspiring student possesses them or not. Sometimes, the students are fundamentally incapable of meeting the demands.

Skill and Efficiency

Every occupation requires one or the other kind of skill for efficiency. Sometimes, the occupational choice by a student may not have this as a consideration. For example, a student who is weak in mathematics may choose engineering as a career.

Personality Makeup

A reserved or shy person generally does not make a successful salesman. So the student has to take into account his/her personality makeup also for making an occupational choice. An individual who has no sympathy for people in trouble may not make a good doctor or social worker.

Physical Strength and Stamina

Those who want to become professional sports persons may require it, as also a student with an ambition to become an officer in the army.

Choosing an Occupation on the Influence of Others

Family has the unique distinction of making two kinds of influences on an individual. Biological influence on an individual determines his/her potential, personality, physique, and sociopsychological influence which make him/her give undue preference. An individual from a lower socioeconomic family with poor education may find it more realistic to think of lowly placed semiskilled or unskilled jobs.

Friends and Acquaintances

A young student is likely to come under the influence of close family members such as an uncle, an aunt, and a cousin and take their occupation as his/her model occupation. Similarly, friends and seniors in the college also influence in choosing a career.

Lack of Information on Career Option and Training

Mistakes in choice of occupation also occur due to the lack of information on career option and training.

Vocational Guidance Programs in Schools

The aims of vocational program are to:

- Help students know their general and specific abilities and skills in relation to the occupation under consideration
- Make available information regarding technical knowledge and skills that are prerequisites for success in an occupation
- Help students understand the characteristics of an occupation
- Enable students to develop their points of view regarding the choice of an occupation
- Provide information regarding financial aids to students and to enable them to pursue their occupational choice.

Vocational Guidance Techniques

- *Career corner:* An occupational information corner is set up for making the occupational information easily accessible to the students.
- The literature on occupational information is displayed which will help the students' free access to literature.
- *Career displays:* Newspaper cuttings and advertisements are used to give an idea of the current occupational scenario. Displays are also used to direct students to the source of further assistance such as library, guidance worker, teacher, and prospective employer.

- *Career talks:* Talks on courses, training programs, occupation, occupational structure, and career planning are organized for students.
- *Career conference:* Weekly, monthly, and half-yearly events/conferences are organized to attract the students, covering several occupations together. The parents are also invited since they generally are an influencing force in the occupational choice of children.
- *Career exhibition:* Occupational information is made available to students through organizing an exhibition. Exhibitions are an effective means of orienting motivating students toward occupations.

CONCLUSION

To ensure mental well being of students, it is recommended that all schools have trained counselors for guidance. In the absence of school counselors, teachers have a major role in providing guidance for common behavioral problems and helping students to make vocational choices. Schools should organise vocational programs and fairs at regular intervals for higher secondary school students to enable informed career choices.

SUGGESTED READING

1. Darakhshan P, Shameem A. The Role of Guidance and Counseling in Schools: A Literature Review. International Journal of Indian Psychology. 2023:11;558-68.
2. Galagali PM, Luiz N. School performance in adolescence. In: Pemde H, Ratna Kumari TL, Galagali PM, Velmurugan (Eds). Adolescent Friendly Pediatric Practice. New Delhi: Jaypee Brothers Medical Publishers; 2024. pp. 225-36.
3. Yuen, M. Exploring Hong Kong Chinese guidance teachers' positive beliefs: A focus group study. International Journal for the Advancement of Counseling. 2002:24;169-82.

20 CHAPTER

Life Skills Education

Anuradha HS

INTRODUCTION

Life skills are the most important tool for helping youth to act in a responsible manner, make informed decisions about their health and well-being, and develop self-efficacy and control over their lives. Young people today feel more challenged than ever in the face of peer pressure, social media, and unrealistic expectations from society. It is clearly becoming evident that only life skills offer the unshakeable foundation for them to overcome and rise above these challenges.

WHAT ARE LIFE SKILLS?

The World Health Organization (WHO) has defined life skills as "The abilities for adaptive and positive behavior that enable individuals to deal effectively with the demands and challenges of everyday life".

Adaptive behavior means having the flexibility and resilience to overcome challenges. Positive behavior is having the ability to focus on possibilities rather than give up in the face of difficulties and conflict. Ten core life skills have been given by the WHO **(Box 1)**.

BOX 1: World Health Organization's 10 core life skills.

1. Self-awareness
2. Empathy
3. Critical thinking
4. Creative thinking
5. Decision-making
6. Problem-solving
7. Effective communication
8. Interpersonal relationships
9. Coping with stress
10. Coping with emotions

IMPORTANCE OF LIFE SKILLS IN ADOLESCENCE

Life skills education for adolescents is crucial in equipping them with the essential tools and knowledge needed to navigate the challenges of adolescence and prepare for the complexities of adulthood. In light of alarming statistics related to mental health, substance abuse, and bullying, the need for a comprehensive life skills curriculum becomes even more apparent. There are several reasons, however, that make life skill education imperative in adolescence:

1. *Mental health challenges:* The impact of the COVID-19 pandemic on adolescents' mental health cannot be underestimated. A staggering 37% of high school students reported experiencing adverse mental health symptoms during this period, with 44% indicating signs of depression within the last year. According to a National Institute on Mental Illness (NAMI) poll, 64% of teens believe that the world is more stressful now than when their parents were their age. Academic pressures, social expectations, and the influence of social media contribute significantly to these distressing statistics.
2. *Substance abuse concerns:* The escalating issue of substance abuse, encompassing both alcohol and drug use, poses a significant concern among adolescents. Alarming statistics indicate that a minimum of one in eight teenagers engaged in the misuse of illicit substances within the last year. Notably, key findings reveal a 61% surge in drug use among eighth graders between 2016 and 2020, coupled with a concerning admission of alcohol abuse by 62% of twelfth-grade teenagers. This disturbing trend, where half of adolescents have misused drugs at least once, underscores the imperative for prompt intervention and educational initiatives.
3. *Prevalence of bullying and cyberbullying:* The pervasive issue of bullying and cyberbullying has garnered attention on a global scale. Parental reports indicate that the highest incidence of cyberbullying is observed in India, where 37% of parents acknowledge their children encountering online harassment, as revealed by Statista. In European countries, namely, Denmark, Finland, the Netherlands, and Norway, children face heightened risks of online sexual exploitation and exposure to

harmful content, as highlighted by the European Parliament. Shockingly, one in every five students (20.2%) reports being bullied, emphasizing the widespread nature of this problem according to the National Center for Educational Statistics in 2019. Additionally, a notable 49.8% of tweens aged 9–12 years old disclosed experiencing bullying at school, with 14.5% revealing instances of online bullying, according to research by Patchin and Hinduja in 2020.

4. *Adolescent development:* In times to come, teens will face choices around screen time, social media, friendships, behavior, motivation, and resilience. But the biggest challenge they face is figuring out who they really are and accepting themselves. In these years, they ask themselves three big questions:
   a. "Who am I?" which is about finding their own identity
   b. "Do I like myself?" which is about feeling good about who they are
   c. "Will I be okay in my future?" which is about worrying if things will work out as they grow up.

   By learning life skills, teenagers can handle all these big questions and challenges during this time.
5. *Academic pressure:* The impact of academic pressure on children's well-being requires careful attention from health experts and researchers focusing on child development. Supported by firsthand experiences of young individuals, previous research indicates that academic pressure encompasses factors such as the "fear of failure, worries about the future, persistent stress related to workload and exams, concerns about parental expectations, and the competition with peers for grades". The root causes of this pressure are complex, but a life skill approach is the best solution for this.
6. *Sexual and reproductive health:* Sexual and reproductive health in adolescents is a crucial aspect of their overall well-being. Providing life skills education to adolescents is directly linked to promoting responsible behavior, informed decision-making, and healthy relationships. Life skills education equips adolescents with the knowledge and skills needed to navigate issues related to sexual and reproductive health, such as understanding their

bodies, making informed choices, and practicing safe behaviors. It also addresses communication skills, self-awareness, and building respectful relationships, fostering a foundation for a positive and informed approach to sexual and reproductive health throughout their lives. In 31 of 36 countries with available data, <50% of married adolescent girls make informed decisions regarding sexual relations, contraceptive use, and reproductive health. Sexual behavior plays a major role in preventing teen pregnancy and sexually transmitted diseases (STDs), and sexual behavior in turn is directly linked to life skills.

7. *Health and hygiene:* Health and hygiene play a crucial role in the well-being of adolescents, influencing both their physical and mental development. Life skills education is intricately connected to this aspect of their lives. Adolescents who receive comprehensive life skills education are equipped with the knowledge and skills needed to maintain good health and hygiene practices. This education covers essential topics such as personal hygiene, nutrition, exercise, and mental well-being. By instilling these life skills, adolescents can make informed decisions about their health, cultivate positive habits, and develop a strong foundation for a healthy lifestyle that extends into adulthood.

Imparting Life Skills in Office Practice

Imparting effective life skills education to adolescents can be done through a combination of individual and group formats and either online or offline.

All counselors have this unique opportunity to provide life skill education to adolescents in their office. Life skill education can be imparted in two different ways: Either one-on-one or in a group. Parents can also be included in the process to initiate lifestyle modification and foster positive behaviors.

Individual Format for Life Skill Education

- *Personalized goal setting:* Counselors can work with each adolescent to identify personal goals, both short-term and long-term, and help them break down goals into achievable steps.

HEADSSS or SSHADES is a tool for psychosocial assessment of an adolescent. It is an acronym that stands for Home, Education/Employment, Eating, Activities, Drugs, Sexuality, Suicidal ideation, and Safety. It is very useful in identifying the adolescent's strengths and weaknesses and teach life skills that will steer them toward informed decision-making and develop emotional resilience. The different ways in which life skills can be taught are as follows.

- *Self-awareness exercises:* To promote self-reflection and self-awareness. Encourage journaling or mindfulness practices to enhance emotional intelligence.
- *Time-management skills:* They can teach effective time-management techniques, such as creating schedules and setting priorities. They also help them understand the importance of balancing responsibilities and leisure.
- *Career exploration:* Counseling sessions can be used to conduct one-on-one discussions about career interests and potential paths. Counselors can offer information about different professions, educational requirements, and career planning.
- *Communication skills:* Adolescents can be taught to focus on improving verbal and written communication skills, practice active listening, and learn effective ways to express thoughts and feelings.
- *Stress management techniques:* Adolescent stress is the root cause of many physical and mental health issues, and introducing stress-reducing strategies such as deep breathing, meditation, or exercise helps them to understand the importance of recognizing and managing stress in a healthy way.

LIFE SKILLS IN GROUP FORMAT

Imparting effective life skills education to adolescents can be done through a combination of individual and group formats, but online mode is particularly effective for group coaching sessions. Group life skill education can be used in the following ways:

- *Team-building activities:* Get adolescents involved in team activities to build teamwork and cooperation. This helps them feel connected and supported.

- *Conflict resolution workshops:* Hold workshops on peacefully resolving conflicts and understanding different points of view. Encourage open communication and empathy to prevent and handle bullying.
- *Peer learning sessions:* Facilitate discussions where adolescents can share experiences and learn from each other. Create a supportive environment for peer mentoring.
- *Role-playing exercises:* Use role-playing to simulate real-life scenarios, enhancing problem-solving and decision-making skills. Focus on situations related to relationships, peer pressure, and communication challenges.
- *Leadership development:* Provide chances for group members to take on leadership roles. Develop skills such as delegation, motivation, and effective decision-making.
- *Community engagement:* Organize activities that involve the group in community service or projects and encourage a sense of responsibility and social awareness.
- *Digital know-how:* Conduct workshops on digital literacy covering online safety, responsible social media use, and digital citizenship. Discuss the impact of technology on mental health.
- *Culture appreciation:* Promote understanding and appreciation of cultural diversity through dedicated sessions.

LIFE SKILLS EDUCATION IN SCHOOL

The most impactful and cost-effective way of giving life skill education to teens has been in a school setting. Schools worldwide have used life skills as a successful intervention in creating a healthy school environment and addressed key modifiable risk factors such as smoking, alcohol, tobacco, nutrition, and physical activity responsible for noncommunicable diseases, which are a major health concern today. Both traditional bullying and cyberbullying are another space where life skills such as interpersonal communication, empathy, and self-awareness have proved to be a game changer.

An example of a successful life skill education program is CDC's (Centers for Disease Control and Prevention) DASH (Division of Adolescent and School Health) program that is focused on establishing healthy youth behavior and prevention of human immunodeficiency virus (HIV), STDs, and unintended pregnancy.

CONCLUSION

Life skills education emerges as an indispensable cornerstone in fostering holistic adolescent development. The transformative impact extends beyond individual growth, creating a ripple effect within communities as adolescents, armed with newfound competencies, become catalysts for positive change.

SUGGESTED READING

1. Division of Adolescent and School Health. (2024). National Center for Chronic Disease Prevention and Health Promotion. [online] Available from https://www.cdc.gov/healthyyouth/about/index.htm#anchor_1598380154 [Last accessed September, 2024].
2. Nair MKC, Bhattacharya P, Toshniwal S. Anticipatory guidance in adolescents. In: Kumar RR, Ratageri VH, Gupta P (Eds). IAP In Standard Treatment Guidelines 2022. New Delhi: Jaypee Brothers Medical Publishers; 2023. pp. 920-5.
3. World Health Organization. (2020). Life skills education school handbook: prevention of noncommunicable diseases. [online] Available from https://www.who.int/publications/i/item/9789240005020 [Last accessed September, 2024].

21 CHAPTER

Depressive Disorders Among Adolescents

Anil Kumar TV, MKC Nair

INTRODUCTION

Depression, once thought to be a disease of adults, is no more considered rare in children (2–4%) and adolescents (4–8%). Depressive disorders—major depressive disorder (unipolar depression), dysthymic disorder (chronic, mild depression), and bipolar disorder (manic depression)—can have far-reaching effects on the functioning and adjustment of young people. Among both children and adolescents, depressive disorders confer an increased risk for illness and interpersonal and psychosocial difficulties that persist long after the depressive episode is resolved. In adolescents, there is also an increased risk for substance abuse and suicidal behavior. Unfortunately, these disorders often go unrecognized by families and physicians alike. Signs of depressive disorders in young people often are viewed as normal mood swings typical of a particular developmental stage. In addition, healthcare professionals may be reluctant to prematurely "label" a young person with a mental illness diagnosis. Yet early diagnosis and treatment of depressive disorders are critical to healthy emotional, social, and behavioral development. There has been a marked increase in adolescent depression and anxiety post COVID-19.

Depression subsequently results in poor scholastic performance, psychological problems, substance abuse, and even suicide. A majority of them approach the pediatrician or the general practitioner with vague so-called functional symptoms. A recent change in behavior with sad or irritable mood lasting for >2 weeks indicates a depression. The same criteria for adults are used for diagnosing depression in children. But we may not get a typical adult type of depressive features in children, as clinical presentation varies according to the developmental stage of the child.

UNDERSTANDING DEPRESSION—BECK'S COGNITIVE THEORY

Beck hypothesized that the cognitive symptoms of depression may often precede affective or mood symptoms; that is, if you think you are ugly or that if you are a failure, it would not be surprising if those thoughts lead to a depressed mood. According to Beck, it is these negative cognitions that are central to depression rather than, for example, the low rates of reinforcement postulated by the behavioral view. There are underlying depressogenic schemas or dysfunctional feelings. These depression-producing feelings develop during childhood and adolescence as a function of one's experiences with one's parents and with significant others (teachers, peers, etc.). Children who lose a parent or who have poor parenting are prone to developing such depressogenic schemas. These schemas or beliefs are thought to serve as the underlying diathesis or vulnerability to develop depression, although they may lay dormant for years in the absence of significant stressors. However, when dysfunctional beliefs are activated by current stressors, the negative cognitive triad becomes apparent and is experienced by the depressed person in the form of negative automatic thoughts. These are thoughts that often occur just below the surface of awareness and that involve unpleasant pessimistic predictions. These pessimistic predictors tend to center on the three themes of the negative triad.

Negative Cognitive Triad

- Negative thoughts about the self as in above mentioned (e.g., I am ugly, I am worthless, I am a failure)
- Negative thoughts about one's experiences and the surrounding (e.g., no one loves me, people treat me badly)
- Negative thoughts about one's future (it is hopeless because things will always be this way).

Beck also postulates that the negative cognitive triad tends to be maintained by a variety of cognitive biases or distortions. These include:

- *Dichotomous or all-or-none reasoning*, which involves a tendency to think in extremes (e.g., If I cannot get it 100% right, there is no point in doing it at all).
- *Selective abstraction*, which involves a tendency to focus on one negative detail of a situation while ignoring the other elements of the situation (e.g., I did not have a moment of pleasure ever; not because this is true but because he/she selectively remembered the negative things and not the positive things).
- *Arbitrary inference*, jumping to a conclusion based on minimal or no evidence (e.g., a depressed person might, after an initial homework assignment from a cognitive therapist did not work, start believing "This therapy will not work for me").
- *Overgeneralization* involves a tendency to draw sweeping conclusions from a single condition or from a single perhaps rather unimportant event (e.g., someone who makes one mistake may conclude "everything I do goes wrong").

Although research supports most features of the discipline aspects of Beck's theory, research directed toward confirming the causal hypothesis has mixed responses.

DEPRESSION IN ADOLESCENCE

Adolescents with depressive illness feel sad and may consistently understand their plight as hopeless. They may not be comforted by relationships with family and friends. Adolescents with a depressive illness will frequently show poor concentration, extreme difficulty in self-starting, and striking changes in thinking and behaving, feel tired and dragged out, and may feel guilty or worthless. Clinical features of adolescent depression are similar to those of adult depression.

- Complains of "feeling sad", "apathetic", "lacking energy".
- Sleep disturbances are more common and there is difficulty getting into sleep or tendency to wake up in between.
- Appetite may be either reduced or increased.

- Bodily preoccupation, worries over his/her appearance or minor health problems.
- Suicidal thoughts are relatively common.

DEPRESSION IN PREADOLESCENCE

- Apathy, verbal and motor retardation, and loss of appetite are the classic features of depression in preadolescence.
- Psychosomatic symptoms (e.g., headache or abdominal pain)
- Poor school performance with poor concentration and attention
- Irritability and social withdrawal
- Sleep and appetite disturbance may be less common.
- Low self-esteem and feeling of "I am not good as compared to others"
- Complains of feeling "bored" and has lack of interest in usual activities.

PREDISPOSING FACTORS

- *Genetic:* Depressive symptoms are higher in family members of seriously depressed children.
- *Biological factors:* There is strong evidence in favor of neurotransmitter (monoamine metabolism) and endocrine abnormalities in depression.
- *Chronic life adversities:* Babies and toddlers who are neglected and deprived of affection are at special risk for developing depression. Depressed children are more likely to come from broken homes and from homes with chronic stresses, for example, parental alcoholism, abuse, and rejection.
- *Temperament:* Quiet children with regular habits and slow to adapt to new experiences are predisposed to emotional disorder.
- *Undesirable life events:* An event at home or at school and experience of loss in previous 12 months are important triggering factors.

ASSESSMENT

Screening: Trivandrum Screening Questionnaire—Mental Health (TSQ-M) and Beck's Depression Inventory (BDI) can be used for screening.

The Diagnostic and Statistical Manual of Mental Disorders, 5th edition (DSM-5) diagnoses a major depressive disorder as a period of at least 2 weeks during which there is a depressed mood or loss of interest or pleasure in almost all activities, plus at least four additional symptoms from a list that include weight changes, sleep disturbances, changes in psychomotor activity, fatigue, feelings of worthlessness or guilt, impaired concentration or decision-making ability, or thoughts of suicide.

- Establish depression—nature, extent, and disability—by interviewing the parent and child and gathering information from school.
- Look for stressors in the school/home.
- *Consider differential diagnosis:*
  - Normal reactive feelings of sadness and unhappiness
  - Physical conditions accompanied by depressed mood change, e.g., hypothyroidism
  - Psychosis (early onset schizophrenia with features like delusions, hallucinations, disorganized speech/behavior, catatonic symptoms, and negative symptoms)
- *Look for comorbidity:*
  - Anxiety disorders seen in 40–60% of patients (separation anxiety disorder, phobia, generalized anxiety disorder)
  - Conduct disorder seen in 20–30% of patients (presenting with aggressive and destructive behavior, deceitfulness, or violation of social rules)
  - Substance abuse (alcohol, smoking, etc.).

DRUG MANAGEMENT

Management of depression involves:

- Drug therapy to correct neurotransmitter defect
- Individual/group counseling to overcome the cognitive error
- Social interventions to support the adolescent at home and school.

Counselors should emphasize the importance of following a healthy lifestyle, balanced nutrition, adequate exercise and sleep, and healthy media use while managing adolescents with depression. Recent research is exploring the various biomarkers in adolescent depression like increase in interleukin-6 and decrease in brain-derived neurotrophic factor (BDNF) for precision diagnosis and management.

Indications for drug use are:

- Severe symptoms
- Patient not responding to psychological treatment alone
- Bipolar depression (children with a history of mania and depression). In bipolar depression, we have to start treatment with mood stabilizers (lithium or sodium valproate) followed by antidepressants, if not showing satisfactory improvement.
- Psychotic symptoms (delusions and hallucinations)
- Chronic recurrent depression.

Tricyclic antidepressants (TCA) are found to be ineffective for the treatment of depression in children in contrast to their use in adults. A number of placebo-controlled clinical trials failed to demonstrate the efficacy of several different TCA medications in depressed children and adolescents. In contrast, selective serotonin reuptake inhibitors (SSRIs) appear to be effective in this age cohort. In a large multisite trial of depressed children and adolescents, fluoxetine was found to be superior to placebo.

Fluoxetine and Sertraline

Commonly used antidepressants are fluoxetine (e.g., Fludac, Prodep, Flunil) available as 20 mg capsules and 20 mg/5 mL liquid preparation. The starting dose is 5 mg taken with breakfast and the dose is increased up to 20 mg. Alternatively, sertraline (e.g., Serta, Serlift) available as 50 mg tablets may be used, with a starting dose of 25 mg in children and 50 mg in adolescents. There are three phases in the management of depression.

Acute Phase

Continue the drug for 4–6 weeks. Define the target symptoms; discuss side effects, dose schedule, and delay of onset of antidepressant action; look for side effects. If the response is inadequate, increase the dose or change the drug.

Continuation Phase

Continue the same dose for 6–12 months along with psychological methods.

Maintenance

Maintenance is done is to prevent recurrence of depression in the following situations: Multiple severe episodes, family history of bipolar disorder or recurrent depressive disorder, comorbid psychotic symptoms, stressful/nonsupportive environment, and residual symptoms.

Resistant Depression

Poor treatment response may be due to the following reasons:
- Inadequate dose, duration, and compliance of drug treatment
- Inadequate psychological intervention
- Presence of comorbid condition—psychotic/medical
- Bipolar depression
- Presence of chronic and severe stressors (e.g., sexual abuse)

Treatment for resistant depression includes optimization of dose and duration, use of a different drug, augmentation with thyroid hormones and mood stabilizers (lithium), electroconvulsive therapy, and patient and family education and support.

COURSE AND OUTCOME OF DEPRESSION

The mean duration of one episode of depression is 7–9 months, and 70–80% of patients recover at the end of 1 year. Good improvement is seen if depression is secondary to a stressor and if we are able to relieve the stress. An increased chance of recurrence is seen in children with early onset and those with a history of previous episodes, comorbid psychotic symptoms, poor drug compliance, negative life events, and positive family history in parents. Twenty to thirty percent of depressive children develop manic episodes (bipolar disorder) on follow-up. Risk factors include early onset, psychotic features, and a positive family history of bipolar disorder.

Cost of depression, if untreated, are poor psychosocial outcome, school failure, recurrent depression, substance use (alcohol, smoking, etc.), and suicide (risk factors—past attempts, family history of suicide, history of family violence, abuse, impulsivity, and availability of lethal agents).

WHEN TO REFER TO A PSYCHIATRIST

Depression, a common childhood and adolescent problem, can be identified and effectively managed by pediatricians. Only those children who require expert evaluation and management may be referred to a psychiatrist. Referral is also indicated if there is no response or worsening, high risk of suicide, relapses of symptoms, atypical features, psychotic features of delusion and hallucination, and associated substance abuse.

INDIVIDUAL/GROUP COUNSELING

A supportive relationship with the therapist is very important. Patient and family education regarding the nature of the illness, complication, and the need for treatment is the first step. Efforts should be taken to alleviate any stressors that are identified during assessment as the presence of stressors is known to worsen the prognosis. Cognitive therapy methods are useful in correcting a defective thinking process, which results in depressed mood. Cognitive behavioral therapy (CBT) is indicated to overcome the cognitive error arising out of a defective thought process.

- *Cognitive error:* Overgeneralization, maximization of negative and minimization of positive attributes of the person.
- *Thought process:* Irrational, illogical, and unrealistic.

Although drug therapy is a must for a severe and extreme form of depression, often supported by individual counseling sessions, the large majority of mild and moderate depression identified in schools or similar situations needs only a group counseling approach. Building self-esteem of the adolescent is an important step in correcting the cognitive error.

Building Self-esteem

- *Step 1: Procedure:* Ask all the students to write the heading *"good qualities in me"* on one side of the paper and *"bad qualities in me"* on the other side and then announce: "*write all your good qualities, abilities—physical or mental—everything good in you, under the heading 'good qualities in me'*". Give 3 minutes, and ask all the students to write as much as they can; after 3 minutes, give a sign to stop. "*Now turn and write all your bad qualities in 3 minutes time, this could be your bad habits, drawbacks, anything you feel uncomfortable about yourself*". After 3 minutes, "stop".

- *Step 2: Sharing in small groups:* Divide the class into small groups of three or four and discuss. Which one was easy? To write down good qualities or noting down the bad qualities? How many good qualities could be listed? Does the number of bad qualities exceed the number of good qualities? Why?

Ask them to read out what they have written in the small group. What was your feeling when you read your good qualities and bad qualities?

Help them to share their insight from this exercise as done in the small group. Most often, we find it difficult to recognize the good qualities in us and are uncomfortable to talk about them. We may make a long list of bad qualities in ourselves as well as in others, but the lists of virtues are always too short. Why is it so? Why do we always stress the negative points?

This is because we always think negatively about ourselves and find ourselves worthless. To understand this, you have to know about the self-image each one is carrying with oneself. This falls into three categories.

Negative Self-esteem or Inferiority Complex

If a person thinks he is inadequate and views himself as a failure, he is having a negative self-image. He thinks himself worthless, unable to face problems and situations. This self-talk makes him feel inferior to everybody and his behavior will be destructive. He will:

- Avoid problematic situations
- Curse himself always
- Be jealous of others' abilities
- Be dissatisfied
- Ridicule and criticize others as he considers them worthless
- Feel lonely because he thinks that nobody loves him

- Have a sense of insecurity, restlessness, and depression
- Compare himself with others and confirm that he is inferior to them.

High Self-esteem (Pride)

It is as destructive as low self-esteem. A person with high self-esteem praises himself and believes that he is one step above others; he has no self-awareness, he will praise himself and show manipulative behavior to make others praise him, he never accepts his shortcomings, he will be selfish all the time, and he will feel insecure and restless. Both these categories of people have no self-awareness, do not accept themselves, and, therefore, cannot accept others.

Positive Self-image (Strong Self-esteem)

This is the healthy attitude. A person with strong self-esteem understands and accepts himself. He knows his capabilities and shortcomings and likes to be himself. He will not compare himself with others and brood on the qualities lacking in him. He will have courage and internal security. He finds the virtues in others and accepts them. He leads a creative life.

Our mental health is dependent on our self-image. One who considers himself inadequate, insecure, and a failure becomes a criminal or psychiatric patient. We have to accept others. It is possible only when we know our capabilities and shortcomings and accept ourselves. A person who cannot accept himself thinks and acts negatively always, and this will become a self-fulfilling prophecy. The reason is this—when he hates himself, he expects others also to hate him. Therefore, his acts and behavior will be in such a way to make others hate him. Then he confirms his idea—"what I thought is true".

Strong self-esteem is essential for healthy interpersonal relationships. When we expose ourselves—our abilities and shortcomings—to others, they understand and accept us. And vice versa also should happen, because if we do not know about a person, we cannot accept him. If we do not have self-esteem and self-awareness, we cannot present ourselves in the company of others. So, this becomes a vicious circle.

CONCLUSION

Adolescent depression can clinically present as a recent decline in academic performance, psychosomatic problems, extreme anger issues and/or withdrawal with impaired functioning at home, school and social circles. If untreated, it can lead to drug use and suicidal behavior. Mild to moderate cases of depression can be managed with counseling and cognitive behavior therapy. Severe cases of depression require pharmacotherapy in addition. Regular follow ups are recommended for evaluating response to therapy and remission.

SUGGESTED READING

1. American Psychiatric Association. Diagnostic and Statistical Manual of Mental Disorders, 5th edition. Arlington, TX: American Psychiatric Publishing; 2013.
2. Grover S, Avasthi A. Clinical practice guidelines for the management of depression in children and adolescents. Indian J Psychiatry. 2019;61(Suppl 2):226-40.
3. Hu S, Li X, Yang L. Effects of physical activity in child and adolescent depression and anxiety: role of inflammatory cytokines and stress-related peptide hormones. Front Neurosci. 2023;17:1234409.
4. Panchal U, Salazar de Pablo G, Franco M, Moreno C, Parellada M, Arango C, et al. The impact of COVID-19 lockdown on child and adolescent mental health: systematic review. Eur Child Adolesc Psychiatry. 2023;32:1151-77.
5. Valkenburg PM, Meier A, Beyens I. Social media use and its impact on adolescent mental health: an umbrella review of the evidence. Curr Opin Psychol. 2022;44:58-68.
6. Zielińska M, Łuszczki E, Michońska I, Dereń K. The Mediterranean diet and the Western diet in adolescent depression—current reports. Nutrients. 2022;14(20):4390.
7. Zwolińska W, Dmitrzak-Węglarz M, Słopień A. Biomarkers in child and adolescent depression. Child Psychiatry Hum Dev. 2023;54:266-81.

22 CHAPTER

Perspectives in Family Counseling

Fr MK George SJ, Susha Janardanan

INTRODUCTION

Family is the most important unit of our social fabric and it is a universal social institution. From time immemorial, one or other form of family has existed. While, traditionally, families have played a large number of functions, in a contemporary society, they seem to play fewer roles. The basic functions of a family are providing survival and security, affection, a balance between dependency and autonomy, socially acceptable sexuality training, and creative development of the adolescent child.

CRISIS IN FAMILIES

A contemporary family is characterized by a series of crisis, crisis in relationship, communication, structure, and so on. Joint families are fast breaking up. Nuclear families find the strain of living in the modern world unbearable. Gender relations are becoming more strained, women demand more freedom, domestic violence is on the increase, children are abused, and spouses find their relationships less satisfying. In short, families are in serious trouble and the most vulnerable partaker of the whole drama obviously is the adolescent child. The psychological and social trauma of the child is indeed very severe. It is here that the adolescent pediatrician/child psychologist/counselor, who is expected to have a sound knowledge about "adolescence" itself and reasonable skill in handling adolescents in crisis, is called to identify the source of stress, in apparently normal, broken, or disturbed families.

Instability Factors in Families

- Reduced family functions
- Less kinship orientation

- Wife less dependent
- Decline in economic cooperation
- Overemphasis of the individual
- Decline in the legal opposition to divorce.

Stability Factors in Families

- Careful selection of mates
- Marriage counseling—professional help
- Increasing income—economic security
- Increasing education—education on values, norms, and disciplined way of life can contribute to stability.

Common Problems Faced by Families Today

- *Economic:* Unemployment and underemployment and hence economic insecurity; lack of income leading to debts, depression, long separation of spouses, my money-your money conflict
- *Relational:* Problems vary from simple disagreement to major strife—overdominance by one spouse, clash among children or with neighbors, inability to communicate properly, lack of time together, sexual inadequacies, problems with in-laws, lack of understanding, jealousy, and new family culture.
- *Treatment-related:* Chronic illness among family members
- *Parenting-related:* Lack of skills, ineffective ways of handling children, dual working parents, adjustment problems
- *Psychological:* Inferiority, irresponsibility of spouses, wife beating, premarital and extramarital sex, ego problems, etc.
- *Lifestyle-related:* Intergenerational problems, gambling
- *Sociocultural:* Alcoholism, dowry, suicides, and divorce.

FAMILY COUNSELING

Family counseling is a practice or activity being developed to help those families *who are hurting overtly or covertly*. It is a process through which a family as a whole is enabled to change its patterns of interaction so that all members get some relief, *feel less pain*, and become freer to develop in the direction most satisfying to them. 90% of problems in the family are created by styles of interaction, lack of interaction, or the quality of interaction among family members. Family counseling helps family members find constructive ways to help one another. It focuses on people's families and other relationships; sharing and respecting individuals' different perspectives, beliefs, views, and stories; and exploring possible ways forward. Family counseling can bring about changes not only in individuals but also in their relationships in the family and beyond. In short, family counseling supports children, young people, and adults in difficult situations or those important to them.

Theoretical Models

Different theoretical models exist in family counseling. A therapist may work from a behavioral stance, from Gestalt principles, or from a combination of therapeutic approaches. Whatever the approach, the main goal continues to be to improve the relationship of each family member with the others, so that the family progresses as a harmonious unit. The basic attitudes in family counseling are that family is important for the survival of society, family should be viewed as a system, malfunctioning families can be helped, and ethical and moral dimensions are essential for the survival of the family.

Goals of Family Counseling

- Improved communication among the family members
- Focusing on the relationship rather than on the symptoms
- Mutual need satisfaction
- Nourishing self-esteem
- Providing better opportunities for growth
- Being open to supportive relationships
- Self-actualization, as an ultimate goal.

Steps in Family Counseling

Most family therapists follow steps similar to the ones listed below:

- *Initial information gathering and assessment of the problem:* This will come at the end of all tests which negate any definite physical causes for the symptom. It would mean picking up hints that fall from the lips and gestures of the parents.

- *Defining the problem:* This is likely to take time and require quite intricate skills. However, an alert counselor/pediatrician with wide-open ears and eyes can identify and define the problem.
- *Developing a contract between the counselor/doctor and the family:* The moment the counselor/pediatrician identifies the problem as originating from a defective family system, he/she needs to develop a contract with the family to work on the problem from a psychological perspective.
- *Further data gathering and assessment:* Quite often, initial data are correlated with, added to, reduced, and so on. Hence, a pediatrician/counselor needs to be very alert to gather further data and arrive at a sharper and more accurate definition of the problem.
- *Choosing a plan of intervention:* At this stage, the pediatrician/counselor persuades the family to adapt a planned intervention with a view to solve the problems of the child.
- *Intervening for problem alleviation:* The pediatrician/counselor may even need to intervene for the alleviation of the problem, within the limits of his/her professional practice.
- *Stabilizing the results of the change effort:* Family counseling efforts are not one-shot enterprises. They require patience and time and the results need to be stabilized.
- *Terminating:* Once the results of the counseling processes are stabilized, the counselor can terminate the process, with an assurance to stand by or support in cases of future needs.

System Approaches to Families in Family Counseling

It is noted that every type of problem has a relationship element in it. One person in a family cannot experience a difficulty without it having some effect on other family members. Some difficulties appear as a part of the relationships, like divorce, whereas other difficulties occur because of unexpected events like illness. Whatever the origin of the problem, in order to deal with it effectively, some change will need to occur within the family.

To appreciate how families make these changes, it is important to understand the functioning of family as a system and to place this within the context of the developmental process. The counselor has to consider family as a whole while helping a member of the family, emphasizing factors such as structure, relationship, and communication pattern rather than traits and symptoms of the individual member. Problems are treated by changing the way the system works rather than trying to fix a specific member.

Basic Skills in Family Counseling

Families need to cope with the daily problems of living, face up to the challenges of development, and provide for the emotional needs of their members. Hence, the family counselor has the task of assisting the family in communicating about the meaning they ascribe to their problems. He/she will be looking to identify those areas where they have a shared view and those in which they are in conflict. As the meanings are revealed, the basis for moving toward negotiations for solutions becomes a possibility. For this, the counselor needs to employ several skills and techniques:

- Attending skills
- Listening skills
- Observation skills
- Diagnostic skills
- Responding skills
- Empathetic understanding
- Concreteness
- Self-exploration
- Integrating understanding
- Confrontation
- Summarizing
- Interpretation
- Focusing
- Supporting/modeling behavior
- Facilitating action for change.

Attending skills are availability, relaxed body posture, physical openness, slight forward lean, good eye contact, appropriate facial expression, use of head nods, and hearing vocal messages. The tone, speed and pitch, and listening skills are active listening, empathetic, internal frame of reference, understanding clients on their own, and paying attention to verbal, vocal, and bodily messages.

Tools/Techniques in Family Counseling

Structural Model

- Direct teaching
- *Structural diagram:* When the client talks, the counselor draws a picture of the structures—authority structure, communication structure, and interaction structure—to give an idea to the client how his/her family system works.
- *Paradoxical suggestion:* When the client says it is extremely difficult to continue the relationship, then the counselor can say ... "OK then I will help you to get a divorce, what do you say?" "Then the client will say, "No, no I did not mean it".
- *Role-playing:* Tell the husband and wife to reverse the roles and say the same things they have said to each other; ask them what they felt, and whether they liked it or not coming from the partner.
- *Parent-adult-child model:* Make a contract to improve the situation. It should be simple, practical, and direct. For example, "From tomorrow I will not get angry with my wife for whatever she says. I will listen, then say something, whatever happens, then make it a habit to improve the situation". Get the feedback and then work onto it.

Communication Model

- Analysis of communication pattern, who initiates it, and the channel of communication. This channel may be operating through children.
- Congruence in communication or the matching of what you think and say. In other words, whether you are able to communicate what you think.
- Clarification of communication patterns
- Communication style may be authoritarian, democratic, and *laissez,* meaning "just anyway", not simply bothered.

Humanistic/Right Brain Approach

- *Active imagination:* Imagining the situation to improve the situation, for example, "If we were not fighting, what would we do?" So, when in a stress situation, think in that way and reduce the strife. After sometime, what we visualize becomes part of our behavior. Fantasy is being used.

- *Story-parable-dreams:* Proverbs, for example, "When I see you, I remember the story of ... a story from the Bible, the *Bhagavad Gita*, etc."
- *Reframing:* When he comes, he gets irritated, but when children are present, then he will not react in that way. So by reframing circumstances, situations can improve.
- *Jokes, ambiguities, quotes, aphorisms* (wisdom saying)
- *Creative memory:* Old memories and good moments shared together
- *Action imperative:* There are certain situations where things have to be done in a particular way only to save the family crisis. Identify those situations and make the client understand and do accordingly, like the husband always coming late is a problem. So either the husband has to come early or the wife has to realize that he will come late only, to improve the home situation.
- *Affirmation:* Affirming the right things they are already doing by giving clear messages ... "Yes, you are doing the right thing".
- *Play:* Do what both like to do, like playing together—shuttle, going to beach, and walking together, to awaken the child in you, not necessarily always leading to sex.

Role of Pediatrician in Family Counseling

Counseling a family is a complex activity and someone who wishes to counsel the family is well advised to undertake specialized training in family therapy. Family counseling is a process through which a family as a whole is enabled to change its pattern of interaction so that all members feel less pain and become freer to develop in the direction most satisfying to them. It is a complex process that requires training and extreme sensitivity. The obvious question is whether the busy, overburdened pediatrician can afford or have the energy to be a family counselor. Most often, the answer is a "no". However, the pediatrician has the responsibility to know the processes and procedures, so that he has the option of at least directing the clients in the right direction.

It will be no surprise to pediatricians that many clinical cases attended to by them are more psychosomatic and psychosocial in origin than being physical. Can the pediatrician hope to become a full-time family counselor? Hardly so, and yet pediatricians need to have basic knowledge of family dynamics and family therapy procedures so that they can meaningfully assist those in trouble. There is no doubt that a substantial number of cases that are reported to the pediatricians are related to family problems. The key question is whether the pediatrician can develop sufficient sensitivity and skills to identify those cases and thus avoid unnecessary medication and hassle to the patient and family. The pediatricians can, with some bit of sensitization and short-term courses, play the role of a family therapist. Of course, it will demand certain commitment on the part of the pediatricians to develop the necessary awareness and skills.

In the final analysis, it is a question of ethics and morality too. The pediatrician, as a physician, has the ethical responsibility to check whether the method that he/she follows will be of benefit to the child patient and the family. The question can still remain. Can our pediatricians, with their existing load of work, afford to be pediatrician-counselors? The final answer is that at least when in doubt, he/she can refer to a family counselor. After all, everyone accepts that medical practice is no more a single person's effort. It is a team effort and much more; it requires a multidisciplinary approach.

CONCLUSION

Family is a social institution. It is currently facing various crises such as relationship issues, communication breakdowns, and domestic violence. Family counseling can address all these issues by improving interaction patterns and relationships within the family. The counselor needs to understand family functioning as a system and address problems through systemic changes. This would enable each family member to attain their optimal potential and ensure appropriate growth and development of children and adolescents in the family in all domains and spheres of life.

SUGGESTED READING

1. Anderson DA. New Approaches to Family Pastoral Care. Minnesota: Fortress Press; 1980.
2. Charles Z. The Practice of Social Work. California: Wardsworth Publishing Company; 1985.
3. Clinebell H. Basic Types of Pastoral Counseling. Nashville: Abingdon Press; 1984.

23 CHAPTER

Premarital and Newly Wed Counseling

MKC Nair, Leena Sumaraj

INTRODUCTION

Marriage is a social institution that ensures the basic needs of humans within a protected and nonthreatening environment. Home is the smallest dynamic unit of society that provides not only the basic needs of food, clothing, shelter, and security but also the emotional needs for love and to be loved. It is the safest outlet for a mutually satisfying sexual relationship. Attributes of values, affection, and tolerance are nurtured in a family environment. Both individuals enter marriage with a lot of fantasy; unfortunately, all expectations are not fulfilled post marriage. Fantasy is colored by previous experiences—our own, that of others', and media projections. Reality may be unexpectedly good or bad and marriage is all about accepting it gracefully. It gives an opportunity for the spouses to grow together, develop love and understanding, and enrich their family life.

MARITAL DISHARMONY

Essentially, marriage is a union of two individuals in wedlock with the objectives of mutually satisfying sexual relationship, enduring companionship, and bringing up children. It is a contract between two individuals of different personalities, taste, outlook, and life experiences. Marital harmony depends on effective communication, mutual understanding and respect, love, affection, and consideration for each other's emotional, social, and economic needs. In spite of our best efforts, marriages do fail and very often the reasons cited are not convincing enough. Hence, a counselor has to take the approach of ruling out serious mental health issues and sexuality issues first, before embarking on a regular counseling schedule.

Mental Health Problems

The primary problem could be an adjustment disorder due to personality factors, mental illness, substance-related disorders, sexual problems, impulse control disorders, and problems related to children and family members. Those with paranoid disorders may be oversensitive, bear grudges persistently, and are suspicious all the time. There is also a group of histrionic personality disorders with self-dramatization, exaggerated expression of emotions, shallow interpersonal relationship, seductive behavior, frigidity, and overconcern for physical appearance. Those with antisocial personality may not have any concern for others, sense of social responsibility, regard for social norms, or enduring relationships. They show low frustration tolerance and impulsiveness, fail to learn from adverse experiences and blame others for their own faults.

Mental illnesses may include minor ones like obsessive-compulsive disorder, specific phobias and anxiety disorders, and major mental illnesses like delusional disorder, schizophrenia, depressive disorder, bipolar disorder, and recurrent depressive disorder. Sexual problems may be the result of sexual abuse in the past or may be just lack of awareness on sexuality dimensions or disorders like sexual desire disorders, sexual arousal disorders, orgasm disorders, sexual pain disorders, sexual disorders due to physical illness, and substance-induced sexual dysfunction. All these disorders may have a medical, psychological, and social background and can cause serious inadequacy in the person leading to marital violence.

Marital Violence

Violence against women in India occurs across her life cycle but more so during adolescence and the reproductive period of youth. Violence and murder because of insufficient dowry are severe and growing threats for women in South Asia. A United Nations Development Programme (UNDP) study in Bangladesh reports "the incidence of physical and verbal abuse of wives due to non-fulfillment of dowry obligations by their fathers is so high that it is almost considered a norm. It occurs in at least 50 percent of recent marriages".

Why Does Marriage Fail?

In spite of all the advantages, marriages do fail nowadays. Once you have ruled out mental health issues, you must think of simple remediable causes. The kind of reasons for divorce petitions registered in Kerala as reported by a popular women's magazine is an eye opener. The reasons cited varied from economic reasons, alcoholism, domestic violence, extramarital relations (both male and female), sexually transmitted diseases, infertility, mental illness, suicidal tendencies, etc. The other significant causes observed included ego problems, inability to get along with the husband's family, the contrast in perceptions about family life, entirely different family backgrounds, differences in socioeconomic status, boys still under the clutches of parents with no independence, nonassertive girls, inability to recognize relatives with ulterior motives, and the capacity and confidence of parents about remarriage. No mention was made about sexual problems, although any practicing marital counselor would know that sexuality-related problems are the number one cause for marital failure.

Although there is a general feeling that the premarital sexual activity is definitely on the rise, a recent United Nations Population Fund (UNFPA)-supported adolescent sexual and reproductive health study conducted at Thiruvananthapuram did not show an alarming picture. About 13.4% of the unmarried had intimate physical contact but none had admitted to having had sexual intercourse. Eleven percent of boys would go for a sexual experience if the opportunity arose. However, the self-admission that 10% of girls and 5% of boys have had sexual abuse in the past was a real eye opener. A recent study conducted by the Nair MKC et al., showed that 97% of adolescent college-going girls, 18–21 years of age, have expressed their resolve to remain as virgin till marriage and the reasons cited were as follows:

- Strongly believe that premarital sex is wrong
- Consider virginity as a sanctified one
- Do not want to cheat future husband
- Do not want to sacrifice virginity just to keep a friend
- Do not want to degrade family
- Do not want to lose self-respect

- Fear that losing virginity will affect marital life
- Do not want to hurt parents
- Do not want to hurt someone for personal pleasure
- Do not want to be cheated (he may not marry me)
- Fear that the person may blackmail in future
- Will be humiliated by the people/society
- Fear of getting pregnant
- Have fear of contracting sexually transmitted infections (STIs) and acquired immunodeficiency syndrome (AIDS)
- Do not have the guts to indulge in sex
- Fear of getting caught (not secure)
- Have not found the right person
- Did not get the right opportunity

It may be noted that only one-fifth of adolescent girls cited fear of pregnancy, STIs, and AIDS as the reason for premarital sexual abstinence as against nearly 90% quoting traditional values, highlighting the importance of premarital counseling classes emphasizing on coping strategies against social and peer pressure for early sexual activity.

CONFLICTS IN MARRIAGE

Not all marriages fail for the same reason. Nor is there usually one reason for the breakdown of a particular marriage. There are other causes, but not quite as often as those listed above. They are failed expectations or unmet needs; addictions and substance abuse; physical, sexual, or emotional abuse; and lack of conflict resolution skills. Affection leads to possessiveness, possessiveness leads to suspicion, and suspicion leads to conflict.

- *Financial matters:* Take the first role in marital conflicts
- *Roles and responsibilities:* Whose job is it to do the grocery shopping? Whose job is it to discipline children or to make rules or major decisions? Whose job is to clean the clothes? The argument continues.
- *Power struggles:* If one of the partners feels that he/she has to win every argument, it could lead to chronic disagreement and failure of the marriage.

- *Sexual difficulties:* They can arise due to the differences in sexual orientation and preferences between couples. In fact, frequency of sex is at times a source of conflict in a marriage. While it is nice to talk to your partner concerning the positions, experimentation, fantasy, etc., at times, all of these things that are part of the sexuality of the marriage can also be a source of difficulty. Once again, choice becomes a part.
- *Jealousy and possessiveness:* Jealousy and possessiveness arise mainly due to lack of trust and strong feelings of inadequacy and insecurity; of course, a certain amount of jealousy and possessiveness should be there for the betterment of marriage.

Types of Conflicts

Rational Versus Irrational Conflicts

Rational conflicts are those conflicts that arise over realistic differences of opinion about some concrete issue. In other words, partners are disagreeing over something that is real and concrete, for example, disagreement over buying a vehicle. Irrational conflicts, on the other hand, are conflicts based on the eccentricity of an individual. These are conflicts over something that is internal, for example, jealousy and possessiveness.

Overt Versus Covert Conflicts

Overt conflicts are very obvious. They are out in the open like yelling, screaming, fighting, and heated arguments. Covert conflicts are the ones that are not on the surface, the ones that are not talked about. The things that are going on between couples that are unspoken, sexual difficulties, many a time, become covert conflicts.

Acute Versus Chronic Conflicts

Acute conflicts are those short-lived explosive arguments and disagreements that you get into, you solve them, and you get on about your normal business. Chronic conflicts are never satisfactorily resolved and constitute a continuing burden on a relationship. Gender roles, at times, form the basis of chronic conflicts in a relationship. In other words, you never really agree on what it means to be man or woman, husband or wife, father or mother.

Personal Versus Interpersonal Conflicts

A personal conflict is when one of the individuals has something going on within him or her, usually the affairs. The problem can detach the partner emotionally and the other partner would not be aware of what the problem is or was. Unfortunately, it is easy sometimes with disagreements, especially if partners do not have satisfactory resolution skills. It is very easy for disagreements to go from interpersonal to personal.

PREMARITAL COUNSELING—TIPS

In spite of many advantages of premarital counseling, it is still not available to the large majority except for some sections of the Christian community. There are many difficulties in offering the services after the marriage has been fixed and hence anyone above 18 years of age should be offered premarital counseling services. The other practical alternative is to have counseling services for the newly wed couples, which has the great advantage of getting the male partner also. The tips given in the following text, generally useful for premarital counseling, may not be always appropriate for a newly married couple, as they have no more choice on the partner. Hence, the emphasis would always be on the long hard journey toward marital bliss, reserved only for those willing to work toward achieving it.

Qualities of a Good Life Partner

A good life partner will show unconditional acceptance, communicate the love/acceptance, try to perceive/understand difficulties and needs, and try to meet them. An ideal marriage requires maturity, understanding, and a sense of commitment for life from both the partners. Above all, he/she would be someone who tries to protect the partner even against himself/herself, making provision for the family and even for a day when he/she may not be in love anymore. What we need to realize is that instead of branding someone as good or bad, we need to be talking about his/her risk-taking behavior, personal, family, and societal risk. For example, smoking has personal risk, family risk, and societal risk, yet much less as compared with drug addiction.

Why Marry?

To satisfy the need for:

- *Safety and security of home:* Married people can enjoy the warmth and sweetness of a home.
- *Acceptance by partner and society:* Through marriage, an individual gets the acceptance and reputation in the society.
- *Sexual desire without guilt feeling:* It is an avenue for disclosing one's own sexual fantasies and desires.
- *Economic security:* Marriage ensures financial support in case of emergency.
- *Having children:* Strengthens the marital bond when children are born and also adds meaning to life.
- *Companionship in good and bad times:* In marriage, partners are bound to be with each other at times of crisis and trauma.
- *Family unity and societal stability:* Since family is the base of any society, marriage ensures social stability.

The institution of marriage should not be considered as a means of avoiding the nuisance of single status, especially for the female, and to avoid the burden of parents. Some people consider marriage as a mode of treatment for mental illness. However, there is no evidence that mental illness will be cured through marriage and moreover it really becomes a lifelong harassment for the partner and for the family. From the bridegroom's side, family members may take marriage as an easy way out for solving their financial burden. On the other side, a bride is expected to behave appropriately as a wife, as a mother, and as a daughter-in-law. "Where she does not have to be appropriate and be the child again is when she is with her parents. When she is denied that access to her parents, suicide is often the end result".

Compatibility in Marriage

It is always ideal to select a partner from similar social status, educational qualifications, job status, etc.; otherwise, the feeling "if only I had married so and so" may not go from the mind. In traditional arranged marriages, the choice of selection in appearance, complexion, color, and physical build may be limited.

One may not get the ideal partner but lifelong distress can be avoided by being genuine/reasonable in selection. Criteria may not matter much once the couple starts living together lovingly.

Physical Incompatibility

Real or perceived difference in:

- *Height:* Avoid extreme differences, if possible.
- *Complexion:* Black can be beautiful, so need not worry.
- *Obese or thin:* Matching or not is important.
- *Appearance:* Pleasing or not is what matters.
- *Age:* Avoid extreme difference in age.

Psychological Incompatibility

Difference in:

- *Educational status:* Inferiority complex may crop up.
- *Job status:* It creates issues in social gatherings, in an Indian setting.
- *Parental status:* Comparing husband and father is natural but not good.
- *Religion:* Problems in child-rearing issues could crop up later.
- *Personality:* No way of knowing in advance, it is more of a gamble.

Sexual Incompatibility

Most important is the negative thinking and guilt feeling toward sex and sexuality, reinforced by parents and religion and also negative experiences of near and dear ones. If the life partner is also with a similar negative mindset, insensitive to your upbringing, then incompatibility can only worsen.

Physical: We all have a fixed concept of what an ideal couple should be like. Try making oneself more attractive, without sticking to the routines in dressing, and try to compensate inadequacies.

Emotional: The innate nature of a person cannot be changed altogether; hence, enough time should be allowed for the person to evolve. Love is not to be concealed; learn to show it, but what is shown outwardly and what the person basically is should match as she/he can perceive genuineness in day-to-day living.

The Unknown Element

There will always be some special attribute in every person that is silently adored. The partner should to appreciate openly the special quality. Destiny may work beyond imagination; faith in God may help in positive thinking and give inner strength to overcome turmoil.

The best solution to overcome incompatibility is to check incompatibility using Partner Assessment Scale Trivandrum (PAST) (Abridged) and try and make ideal of what one gets.

Partner Assessment Scale Trivandrum (PAST) (For married only) (*Note:* How do you rate yourself in the following domains?)

1. *Reality:* With all the good and bad in marriage overall real-life rating	1. >50%	2. 25–50%	3. <25%
2. *Fantasy:* Fit in with your own fantasy—partner/child/profession	1. >50%	2. 25–50%	3. <25%
3. *Support:* Financial support/family support/peer's support	1. >50%	2. 25–50%	3. <25%
4. *Attitude:* Whether taking the concept of marriage seriously	1. >50%	2. 25–50%	3. <25%
5. *Sexuality:* Sexual satisfaction with husband/wife—overall assessment	1. >50%	2. 25–50%	3. <25%
6. *Personality:* Giving type/abundant (enjoy by giving pleasure to partner)	1. >50%	2. 25–50%	3. <25%
7. *Conflict:* Problems resolved amicably, not getting unduly upset	1. >50%	2. 25–50%	3. <25%

Source: Nair MKC, George B, Mini G. Sexuality counselling for newly-wed couple. In: MKC Nair (Ed). Adolescent Pediatrics, 2nd edition. New Delhi: Nole Vision; 2023; pp. 253-4.)

Adjusting with Partner

Some men are nothing more than grown-up little boys, still looking for mothers, rather than wives. They want someone to minister to their physical needs, keep them well fed and happy, and soothe their egos when they get hurt. Similarly, girls go into marriage with a full-blown image of a man who is nothing short of a person who is rough and tough, strong, and dominant. In such situations, it becomes really tough to build up a healthy relationship. Accept that your partner also partners need to accept each other's fantasies and play up to them. Fantasy may be in personality, dressing style, romantic approach, caring, and being cared. There is no way of knowing early the "real" person, meaning someone who does not wish bad for others as a rule.

Too Good—Good Partner

Someone who genuinely does not want to hurt anybody, wants to keep an image of being good, or is just too much scared to do anything bad

Too Bad—Bad Partner

Someone who does not know how to conceal or does not bother what others think of him/her. Bad qualities overshadow rare goodness.

Reality of Adjustment with Partner

Marriage is coming together of two adult individuals with different personality traits. They might have come from entirely different cultures, roots, upbringings, status, etc. They should not expect that everything to go right straight away. We all enjoy the good qualities of our life partner and at the same time we are bound to accept some bad qualities also. One should have adequate patience, not jumping into conclusions. It is only from experiences that one may understand the person well. We all do hope and wish for a good life partner who understands, cares, shares, loves, and will get along with all the members of the family. Many of the problems, which arise later, have roots in this expectation.

Fantasy apart, in reality, marriages work well if both the partners accept each other as such, respect each other and support each other, share responsibilities for family earning, share household burden, care for children, and neither being a spendthrift nor a miser.

- Do not be in a hurry to mold him/her as you wish, for till now he/she has survived well without the other partner.
- Take care not to publicize the inadequacies.
- Listen to everyone's stories and advice but act only on one's instincts, because no one understands the partner better than the spouse.

- One has a right to your privacy, so has he/she; do not be inquisitive and try to be a detective, for marriage is a mutual game of trust.
- Do not test his/her trust often, for he/she may not accept that one could continue to have affectionate relationships with others.
- All of us are endowed with many good qualities as well as bad qualities, so does our partner.
- Society usually assesses him/her by external appearance and behavior. So keep in mind that only time will enable people to understand the partner better.

Difference between Parents and In-laws

With parents, you assume positive intention in all actions, understand their personality traits, know how to tackle their mood changes, have lots of pleasant memories of the past, and do not have to be appropriate all the time.

Adjustment with In-laws

Appreciate the insecurity of the in-laws; after all, they perceive themselves as the losers, financially, emotionally, and in the power game. Partners should respect in-laws and not precipitate a situation where the partner has to choose between parents and the spouse.

Adjusting with New Family Environment

Partners should try to understand social relationships and the customs and practices of the partner's family, and make all attempts to create a positive image of a kind, caring person, with self-respect and not becoming a doormat at anytime.

Making Marriage Work

Early on in the marriage is the time particularly valuable for couples to build stronger relationships. A person who can understand himself/herself can only understand others. A person who knows his/her capabilities, dreams, hopes, and aspirations can easily understand his/her partner as the same person with all these traits. Marriage will work when one partner or both ignore or avoid the drawbacks of the partner, not because he/she is a fool but because of his/her deep-rooted love toward the partner, accepting him/her as a companion in the journey of life.

Hurting each other physically or emotionally should not be the conflict-resolving strategy. "Inadequacy" of the partner, perceived or real, should not be used against, as a weapon. Thoughts about the fantasy life partner may not die down, but do not rekindle these. In fantasy, the partner may not rate high, but in reality, he/she may be the best. In a successful marriage, partners are usually a major influencer in each other's life inspite of being from different backgrounds and upbringing. Partners should ensure the existence of romance in marriage.

Before Having a Baby—Tips

The ideal age for marriage is between 20 and 30 years, although many are not lucky enough to get the right partner by then.

- Do not delay the first pregnancy.
- Do not forget a medical and gynecological checkup.
- Rule out sexually transmitted diseases.
- Avoid drugs during the second half of menstrual cycle—fertilization occurs around the 14th day.
- Avoid intrauterine infections causing low birth weight, small head, deafness, cataract, various birth defects, etc.
- Toxoplasmosis—avoid partially cooked meat and contact with cat feces by gardening.
- Rubella (German measles)—give MMR vaccination at 15 months of age and rubella vaccine to all teenage girls, to avoid deafness and blindness.

CONCLUSION

- Marriage is a union of two individuals in wedlock with the objectives of mutually satisfying socially acceptable sexual relationship.
- Mental illnesses that affect marital relations may include; anxiety disorders,depressive disorder, bipolar disorder, delusional disorders, obsessive compulsive disorder, specific phobias, etc.

- Marriages fail due to; failed expectations, unmet needs, addictions, physical, sexual, or emotional; or lack of conflict resolution skills.
- Family life education before 18 yrs, premarital counselling above 18 yrs, and newlywed counselling is a feasible strategy to reduce marital conflicts.
- Oath: I am the custodian of my mind, body, and spirit; I will protect , preserve and enhance all three.

SUGGESTED READING

1. Holman TB, Jacquart M. Leisure-activity patterns and marital satisfaction: a further test. Journal of Marriage and the Family. 1988;50(1): 69-77.
2. Leena ML, Nair MKC. Perspectives in Premarital Counselling In: Nair MKC, Leena ML, Russell PS, (Eds). Premarital Health Counselling, 1st edn. Noble Vision (Medical Book Publishers); 2023. pp. 91-103.
3. MKC Nair, Babu G, Mini G. Sexuality counselling for newly-wed couple. In: Nair MKC (Ed). Adolescent Pediatrics, 2nd ed. Noble Vision (Medical Book Publishers); 2023. pp. 247-55.
4. Nair MKC, Thankachi Y, Leena ML, George B, Russell PS. ARSH 3: Reproductive and sexual health knowledge: a comparison among married male and female young adults (15-24 y). Indian J Pediatr. 2013:80(Suppl 2);S203-8.
5. Nair MKC. Early child development—Kerala model. Global Forum for Health Research Forum 3 meeting; 1999; 8-10.
6. Nair MKC. Partner Assessment Scale Trivandrum (PAST). TEENS J Teenage Care Premarital Couns. 2000;1(2).
7. Namboothiri S, Thomas S. Pre-conceptional counselling. In: Nair MKC, Balakrishnan S, (Eds). Handbook of Pediatric & Adolescent Gynecology, 1st edn. Paras Medical Publisher; 2023. pp. 463-76.

24 CHAPTER

Counseling in the Child Rights Perspective

Babu George, MKC Nair

INTRODUCTION

Basic human rights issues include the rights of children (0–18 years); the rights of the vulnerable and the socially disadvantaged have gained significance only recently, even though women's issues had been a subject of discussion since 1975. The United Nations (UN) convention on child rights has, to a certain extent, helped to create awareness regarding child rights and legislations relating to child labor and atrocities against street children. There are many reasons that make children the most vulnerable:

- *Innocence—the hallmark of children*
- *Unawareness that their rights are being violated*
- *Absence of a body to represent their cases*
- *Their inability to fight back making them easy prey for exploitation*
- *The habit of not confiding in someone*
- *The ease with which children can be lured*

This again gets compounded if the child is poor, a girl, from a scheduled tribe/caste, handicapped, or living in remote and inaccessible areas. The issues related to child rights should not be narrowed down to prevention of child labor alone but should also take up the cause of stepchildren, children of nomads, adopted children, victims of terrorism, children of women in jail, child brides, battered children, children in conflict with law, children used for camel racing, children of parents with chronic medical disorders, children of drunkards/alcoholics, and girls in order to ensure that every single child enjoys the "the right to childhood".

As part of propagating awareness on child rights, child book fairs, painting competitions and storytelling workshops for children, and child-to-child programs should be organized, preferably with meaningful youth engagement. Citizens should be made aware of their rights as laid down by the Indian Constitution, and about the existence of various bodies under the government to ensure protection of human rights like the National Human Rights Commission as a remedial action against violation of rights. Protection of rights can be ensured through promotion of equality in development, promotion of unity in diversity, and enforcement of human rights. A charter of child rights should be prepared which should be followed up by a plan of action.

GENDER PERSPECTIVE

Discrimination of a girl child can be in the areas of access to education, quantity and quality of food intake, accessibility to healthcare facilities, and female feticide. Such remarkable differences are not seen in the care of a girl child in Kerala, although subtle discrimination may be noted. The discrimination of a girl child in Kerala, if any, is not family induced but community induced or community ordered, though projected through the family.

In India, girls are subjected to a rigorous disciplining process in families. From the menarche itself, more and more constraints are placed on the freedom allowed for a girl child. They are brought up in a stereotyped role, whereas their experiences outside the house or the influences of satellite television and social media portray the other extreme. Hence, girl children are more pressurized and under dilemma as to what is right and what should be followed.

Unlike boys, girls have a dual role to perform, i.e., of a homemaker as well as a wage earner. Both the social roles have responsibilities, which are at tangent to each other. At home, the girl is expected to obey the male members of the family and portray the role of a nurturing mother or sister, whereas at the workplace, she not only has to work with male members but also has to be assertive in exercising her powers in the job. Demands from family are more for a girl child, right from childhood onward.

As parents are unsure of the girl child's future, right from day 1, savings in the form of gold are kept apart for a girl child. As age increases, dowry or gold is needed to marry off a girl into a respectable family. This dilemma, which the society induces in a girl child's mind knowingly or unknowingly, follows her all through life. In spite of this dilemma, a girl child may have more inner strength than a boy and are better able to face problems in life. The middle class of Indian society, with its hypocrisy and inhibitions, passes down its fears and doubts to children, especially girls.

SEXUALITY ISSUES

"Sex" had been a taboo topic till recently in India. The suppressed sexual libido of men finding its way out as sexual exploitations like pedophilia and rape is another reason for the difficulty that girl children face, when they have to travel or go out after dusk. Family itself is under tremendous pressure due to industrialization and globalization. Commercialism has touched upon every aspect of our life. Alcoholism and the recent trend of families committing suicide due to financial problems, all affect the girl child more than the boy child.

In our country, many people have a distorted idea of sexuality and sensuality. This may be because of the fact that the boys and girls get only the distorted picture of the opposite sex, which is far from the real. The distorted image of a woman/girl that a boys get is more through pornographic books and magazines and much less through direct interactions. Hence, boys are unaware of the aesthetic and spiritual aspect of sex and sexuality. This may also be one of the contributing factors to the difficulty faced by women in going out alone after dusk. Coeducational institutions should be promoted so that boys and girls get an opportunity to understand, respect, and appreciate each other's individuality.

PROTECTING THE EARTH FOR CHILDREN

In the present-day world, children are brought up in such a way that nature is something alien to them. In order to protect the earth, the two types of possible actions are remedial and preventive. It is the duty of parents to provide opportunities for their children to interact with the three elements of nature—water, air, and soil—whereby children will develop the quality of humaneness and empathy, which can be channelized toward protecting the nature. Pollution, poverty, population explosion, and profit motives are the major factors that destroy the earth. Another important problem is the difficulty of human beings in differentiating between little inconveniences in life and crisis in the society. Nature has an order or discipline which if affected will backfire.

Children understand or make sense of the world they live in through the five senses of vision, hearing, touch, smell, and taste. In other words, these five senses form the basis of a child's cognition, which should help the child to reach the height of being able to visualize the unknown. All these are stored in the sixth sense—the mind. Hence, the sixth sense or the mind should be the abode of what is learned and felt rather than just a storehouse of memory.

REACHING THE UNREACHED

Human tendency is to exploit the resources of tomorrow for the pleasure of today. Hence, in the education sector, it is imperative to visualize or foresee the problems of tomorrow and make necessary changes in the present-day education system. There are two types of reaches—the physical reach and the spatial reach. In India, we have been able to attain a better standard of physical reach through universalization of primary education, greater enrollment, and more number of schools in remote areas, but we have not achieved what is called the spatial reach. With regard to spatial reach, we need to answer questions like how long will the children who are in the mainstream of education be there or would continue, what will they gain out of this system of education, are we able to reach them emotionally and intellectually, and how successful they are in life.

Although a quality basic education is every child's fundamental right, there are children who are denied the opportunity for basic education. It is mostly the children from the underprivileged societies who remain unreached by education. Social problems of the tribal and other underprivileged sections of the society need special attention. Another group that is not effectively reached by education is the children with disability. The reason for such children not attending schools may be not only financial constraints but also because of society-induced social and emotional problems. Teachers themselves are unaware of the disability process—impairment leading to disability and causing handicap later on.

CHILD ABUSE AND FAMILY VIOLENCE

Issues of child abuse are gaining importance nowadays because of the increase in the number of cases reported and because of the increasing feeling that the available data on child abuse is nothing but the tip of an iceberg. It is now well known that the abuser is usually a person known to the child and was himself/herself was abused in childhood. The abuse can be either emotional or physical. It is not easy to define abuse. It may range from a milder form to a brutal one. What each person considers as abuse changes from culture to culture. Abuse may range from scolding to severe forms like battering, applying chili powder on bruises and causing burns. In the case of sexually abused young girls, sometimes even less than 10 years of age, the victim continues to be victimized again and again, in the process of getting justice. People look down upon the victim, although she had been in no way responsible for the act and becomes an object of undue attention which is traumatic for her. According to the Protection of Children from Sexual Offences Act (POCSO), all cases of child sexual abuse have to be mandatorily reported to the police.

The major strategies to prevent child abuse would be as follows:

- Parents should always have an eye on every person who is close to the child.
- Children should be sensitized not to allow anybody to touch their private parts or to take liberty with them.
- Make children aware of their rights to protect their body by building life skills.
- This should begin at home itself by allowing children to disagree and to say *no* to matters to which they cannot agree.
- Always be sympathetic toward the victim. Remember this can happen to any child also.
- Parental training for managing children who were abused is needed. Parents should be sensitized on the need for dealing the matter subtly and not by emotional outburst.
- Children, especially girls, should be made aware of the circle of intimacy and personal space that each person can have with them.

- They should also be able to anticipate when the limits will be crossed—whether it is by way of a look, a word, or a touch.
- Parents should not give undue freedom for outsiders inside the home.
- Awareness on the possible legal help available for the victimized is needed.
- More than anything else, parents should anticipate things and deal with situations effectively.
- Parents should not burden the children with knowledge on too much of "would-be-possible" abuse, thus terrorizing them in the process.
- A concerted parent-oriented, teacher-oriented, and society-oriented approach is needed for tackling this issue of child abuse.
- Professional bodies should give counseling to adolescents as a group and make them take an oath:

I am the custodian of my mind, body and spirit.
I will protect them, preserve them and enhance them.

—MKC Nair

CONCLUSION

The fundamental rights of the child need to be nurtured right from birth. These include the right to survival, the right to development, the right to protection and the right to participation. Gender equity should be ensured with equal opportunities for girls and boys to thrive and attain their potential. Any violation of child rights including physical, emotional and sexual abuse and neglect should be handled sensitively by the counselor and reported to the non-abusive caretakers concerned authorities.

SUGGESTED READING

1. Choudhry V, Dayal R, Pillai D, Kalokhe AS, Beier K, Patel V. Child sexual abuse in India: a systematic review. PLoS One. 2018;13:e0205086.
2. Srivastava RN. Right to health for children. Indian Pediatr. 2015;52:15-8.
3. Srinivasan SP, Shruthi S. A comparative review of UNCRC and Indian legislation from the child mental health perspective. Indian J Psychol Med. 2024;46(4):289-97.

25 CHAPTER

Self-counseling

MKC Nair, Shamal Kumar, Deepa Binod

INTRODUCTION

With the limited availability of trained physicians/pediatricians/counselors to deal with psychological problems, self-counseling can be an effective method to help those with mild issues. The prerequisite for an effective self-counseling includes self-awareness, self-motivation, and self-screening.

- Self-awareness is the ability to understand one's own thoughts, feelings, behaviors, and how they impact others and the world around us. It also involves recognizing our strengths and weaknesses, values and beliefs, and how we see ourselves in relation to others.
- Self-motivation is the internal drive that pushes one to take action and achieve our goals without needing external encouragement. It is the ability to find the inner strength to start and continue a task, even when facing challenges.
- Self-screening refers to the process of examining ourselves for potential health/psychological issues or conditions. The goal is to identify potential problems early on, so that early remedial measures could be taken by ourselves.

A successful self-counseling session needs finding strength in not just oneself but also the support system which may include the family and/or friends. Self-counseling is the process of examining one's own behavior, using psychoanalytical methods of: (1) free-thinking, meaning, forming our own opinions and beliefs, rather than just accepting what is officially or commonly believed and taught, and (2) free association meaning, the mental process by which one word or image may spontaneously suggest another without any necessary logical connection. Self-counseling can help one take more effective control of everyday situations and enable to make continued progress (personal growth). Self-counseling takes people on a journey of self-discovery, working at their own pace and in the directions, they most feel comfortable with. However, some problems may be too deep-seated for self-counseling, and these may require additional forms of therapy.

BURDEN OF ANXIETY DISORDERS AND DEPRESSIVE DISORDERS IN INDIA

While all forms of psychosis need assessment by a psychiatrist/clinical psychologist, anxiety disorders, and depressive disorders can be easily diagnosed and managed by an adolescent pediatrician. In a representative sample of 500 adolescents from a rural community in Southern India, who were assessed for the period prevalence of all and specific anxiety disorders using screen for child anxiety related emotional disorders (SCARED) and Beck's depression inventory (BDI), it was reported that:

- The prevalence for all anxiety disorders using the International and Indian SCARED cutoffs was 8.6% and 25.8%, respectively, as against 14.4% for the Diagnostic and Statistical Manual of Mental Disorders, fourth edition, text revision (DSM-IV-TR) criteria.
- Depressive disorders were concurrently present in 23.7% of adolescents with anxiety disorders, and more adolescents with anxiety disorder had multiple mood disorders.
- Depressive disorders were more severe among those with anxiety disorder and the anxiety disorder was more severe in those with depressive disorder.
- As the severity of anxiety disorder increased the severity of the depressive disorders also increased.
- Suicidal behavior was increased by the presence of anxiety disorder, severity of the anxiety disorder, and being a boy also increased the risk.
- Presence of anxiety disorder and comorbid depressive disorder significantly contributed to a risk model for suicidal behavior.

It has become even more important, with the increase in mental health conditions in the post-corona virus disease (COVID) era, as evidenced by systematic review of 15 studies describing 22,996 children/adolescents in India with; behavior/psychological state—79.4%, depression—41.7%, irritability and inattention—42.3%, boredom—35.2%, anxiety—34.5%, significant fear of COVID-19—22.5%, and sleep disturbance—21.3%.

NOORUL ISLAM INSTITUTE OF MEDICAL SCIENCE (NIMS)—CHILD DEVELOPMENT RESEARCH CENTRE–SELF COUNSELING QUESTIONNAIRE

The questionnaire (see **Annexure**) has the following domains:

- Emotional self-awareness (7 Questions)
  Example: Expressing emotion is not easy for me.
- Social self-awareness (7 Questions)
  Example: Care a lot about how I present myself to others.
- Mental health awareness (7 Questions)
  Example: Excess anxiety, sadness, anger, stress affect activities.
- Physical and personal awareness (7 Questions)
  Example: Lazy to do daily exercise as a routine.
- Reproductive health awareness (7 Questions)
  Example: Have infrequent/abnormal menstrual periods.
- Sexual awareness (7 Questions)
  Example: Do you feel uncomfortable discussing sex/sexuality issues.
- Spiritual awareness (7 Questions)
  Example: Use unconditional faith in God to face life problems.
- Partner assessment scale Trivandrum for couples (7 Questions)
  Example: Value system: Both partners share common values.

Ten Commandments for Self-counseling

1. Do not bluff to yourself, though may have to bluff to others sometimes.
2. *You are not God and hence likely to make mistakes:* Take precaution always.
3. *Do not think others have to like you always:* Practice self-love.
4. *Caring and not love:* Trust only the one who cares for you.
5. *Kill enemy by caring when they need your support:* Keep no enmity.

6. *Refuse to take insult:* Replace feeling pathway with cognitive pathway.
7. *Do not think others are lesser than you:* You are also lesser than someone else.
8. *Think of other person's point of view:* Try to be a third party.
9. Do not hurt someone, if possible, do not hurt yourself "ever".
10. I am the custodian of my mind, body, and spirit, I will protect, persevere, and enhance it.

—MKC Nair

SIMPLE SELF-COUNSELING METHODS

Four self-counseling techniques: Meditation, relaxation techniques, free association, and autogenic training. Each of these methods fosters greater self-awareness, emotional regulation, and mental clarity, making them valuable tools in personal development and mental health maintenance.

Meditation

Meditation is a widely practiced cognitive and emotional regulation technique rooted in ancient traditions and supported by contemporary psychological research. It involves training the mind to focus and redirect thoughts, often through breath awareness or guided concentration.

Key forms of meditation applicable to self-counseling include:

- *Mindfulness meditation:* Cultivates nonjudgmental awareness of the present moment. It enhances cognitive flexibility and emotional regulation by allowing individuals to observe their thoughts and feelings without attachment or avoidance.
- *Focused attention meditation:* Centers attention on a single object—commonly the breath, a mantra, or a bodily sensation. This method helps interrupt ruminative thought patterns and improves concentration.
- *Loving-kindness meditation:* Encourages the cultivation of compassion toward oneself and others, thereby supporting emotional healing, particularly in the context of guilt, self-criticism, or interpersonal distress.

Regular meditative practice has been associated with decreased stress reactivity, improved mood, and greater psychological resilience, the key outcomes in effective self-counseling.

Relaxation Techniques

Relaxation techniques are integral to reducing physiological arousal and creating a mental environment conducive to self-reflection. These methods facilitate the downregulation of the autonomic nervous system, counteracting the physiological effects of chronic stress and anxiety. Core relaxation strategies include:

- *Progressive muscle relaxation (PMR):* Involves sequentially tensing and releasing major muscle groups to increase bodily awareness and reduce tension. It enhances somatic mindfulness and can signal psychological readiness for deeper self-exploration.
- *Diaphragmatic breathing:* Also known as deep breathing, it stimulates the parasympathetic nervous system, thereby reducing cortisol levels and inducing calmness.
- *Guided imagery:* Utilizes mental visualization of calming scenes or positive outcomes. It supports emotional regulation and is particularly effective in mitigating anticipatory anxiety.

In the context of self-counseling, relaxation techniques serve both as preparatory tools for introspection and as standalone strategies to manage acute stress responses.

Free Association

Free association, derived from psychoanalytic traditions, is a technique in which individuals articulate their thoughts freely without censorship or logical structuring. This spontaneous expression can be verbal or written and serves to access unconscious material that may be influencing current emotional states or behaviors.

Applications in self-counseling include:

- *Journaling:* Writing continuously and unfiltered for a predetermined period allows the emergence of underlying themes, repressed emotions, and cognitive distortions.

- *Verbal stream-of-consciousness:* Speaking thoughts aloud in a private setting can yield similar benefits, particularly for individuals who process emotions more effectively through auditory expression.

The goal of free association is not immediate problem-solving but rather uncovering of latent content—conflicts, fears, and desires—that may inform future self-guided interventions.

Autogenic Training

Autogenic training, derived from the Greek roots meaning "originating within oneself," is a self-regulation technique that uses verbal cues and guided visualization to elicit a deep relaxation response. This meditation-like practice is centered on the principle that the mind can influence physiological processes through focused, self-directed effort.

The essence of autogenic training lies in learning to consciously command the body to relax. Self-practitioners repeat a series of structured phrases—such as *"My arms are heavy and warm"* or *"My heartbeat is calm and regular"*—while visualizing corresponding bodily sensations. This process systematically induces a state of calm across various parts of the body, leading to reduced sympathetic nervous system activity and enhanced parasympathetic function.

Brain Gym

One of the feasible modes of self-counseling is the Brain Gym Program. It is based on how the brain and body work together and uses easy body movements to help improve learning, focus, memory, and emotional balance. The exercises help both sides of the brain work better as a team, thus helping to improve thinking, reduce stress, better concentration, calmness, and overall brain health.

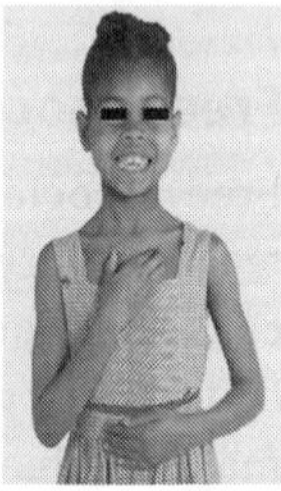

The more commonly used technique is:

THE PACE—stands for *positive, active, clear, and energetic.*

- *Energizer:* Sip the water and hold in the mouth for 10 seconds, breathe regularly and let it in slowly.

- *Brain buttons*: Make a "U" shape with one hand and place your thumb and index finger in the small depressions just below your collarbone, gently press, and rotate in a circular motion. Place the other hand over the navel. Move eyes slowly to the left and right along a horizontal line. Breathe deeply. Change the hands.
- *Cross crawl*: Bring one knee and opposite elbow together. Then bring the other knee and its opposite elbow together. Repeat rhythmically for about 1 minute. This exercise can be done in standing position or sitting position.

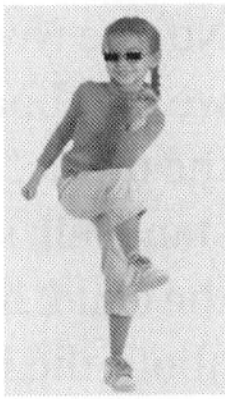

- *Hook ups:*
    - *Part 1*: Cross your ankles. Bring the hand forward and cross and then clasp them together, then bring the hand toward the chest. Breathe deeply allowing the tongue to raise and touch the upper pallet of the mouth.
    - *Part 2*: Place the feet flat on the floor, touch the tip of the fingers together, and then continue to breathe.

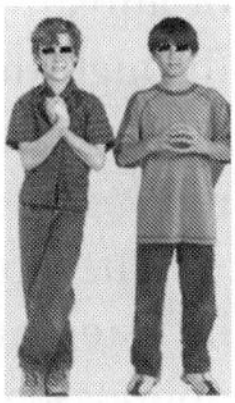

Life Skill Education

Life skills refer to the skills usually associated with managing and living a better quality of life for each one of us, helping to accomplish our ambition, and live to our full potential. Life skills have to merge with life circumstances, culture, beliefs, age, geographic location, etc.

Life skills help one to make informed decisions, communicate effectively, develop coping and self-management skills, and thus help us to lead a healthy and productive life. For adolescents developing appropriate life skills help transit successfully from childhood to adulthood by healthy development of: (1) social emotional skills, (2) social competence, (3) problem solving skills, (4) identify pros and cons of situation, (5) positive social norms and thus avoid abuse of drugs, alcohol, tobacco, etc.

The essential life skills to be considered in self-counseling are: Coping with stress, creative thinking, critical thinking, dealing with emotions, decision making, effective communication, empathy, interpersonal relationship, problem solving capacity, and self-awareness.

SELF-COUNSELING FOR MOTHERS OF CHILDREN WITH AUTISM SPECTRUM DISORDER

No one would contest, if I say that in spite of all supportive services we may boast of, ultimately, it is the mother, who alone have to "face the music." On one side, her whole dream about her child come to a standstill; she does not know how to handle the erratic behaviors of the child; how to face unwanted criticism of people around; worried about the future of the child, and so on. On hearing the diagnosis of autism spectrum disorder (ASD), a good number of them go through the stages of denial, anger, bargaining, depression, and finally acceptance. This process that may take few months could be reduced to few weeks, if only we can initiate self-counseling process.

The mothers of ASD children can practice "self-counseling" skills by listening carefully, asking for clarification, and probing around options that can help most mothers to cope better. The Developmental Pediatrician/Developmental Therapist/Developmental Nurse Counselor managing the ASD child can help the parents learn how to work with emotional conflicts and master the art of healing.

Spiritual Psychology (Hulnick): Spiritual psychology is concerned with the health of the individual's soul and this soul-centered approach believes that "when love is applied to hurt we heal." Practically applied, it helps a person become aware of a recent upset, ride the emotion back in time to the root of the matter (its core), communicate with that portion inside that is fixated, and apply love to it.

CONCLUSION

Many of us practice some "self-counseling" skills innately already. Listening with an open heart, asking for clarification, and probing around options can help most people get better. Further, learning how to work with deep-seated emotional wounds can also be mastered if one learns the proper structure. After all, all it takes is human compassion to heal deeply seated wounds that may have been there for years.

ANNEXURE

Self-counseling

Self-evaluation Questionnaire for Young Adults

I. Emotional self-awareness:

1. Expressing emotion is easy for me.
   1-Often 2-Sometimes 3-Never
2. Do "self-talk" to think about my feelings.
   1-Often 2-Sometimes 3-Never
3. Know what caused my mood change.
   1-Often 2-Sometimes 3-Never
4. Usually aware of my inner emotions.
   1-Often 2-Sometimes 3-Never
5. Like to be alone to think about my feelings.
   1-Often 2-Sometimes 3-Never
6. Think about ways to make myself feel better.
   1-Often 2-Sometimes 3-Never
7. My thinking, feeling, and behavior match.
   1-Often 2-Sometimes 3-Never

II. Social Self-awareness:

8. Care a lot about how I present myself to others.
   1-Often 2-Sometimes 3-Never
9. Easy for me to mingle with others/strangers.
   1-Often 2-Sometimes 3-Never
10. Reasonably concerned about what others think of me.
    1-Often 2-Sometimes 3-Never
11. Do not feel nervous speaking in front of a group.
    1-Often 2-Sometimes 3-Never
12. Step back (in my mind) to examine myself.
    1-Often 2-Sometimes 3-Never
13. Not difficult to work when someone is watching.
    1-Often 2-Sometimes 3-Never
14. Enjoy family time/outings with family.
    1-Often 2-Sometimes 3-Never

III. Mental health

(Note: Feeling anxious, sad, angry/irritable, or stressed/tension at times is normal)

15. Above symptoms out of proportion to cause.
    1-Never 2-Sometimes 3-Often
16. Sleep/appetite/sexual interest affected in the recent past.
    1-Never 2-Sometimes 3-Often
17. Symptoms disturb or affect daily activities.
    1-Never 2-Sometimes 3-Often
18. Feeling that you are good for nothing (worthlessness).
    1-Never 2-Sometimes 3-Often
19. Feeling that there is no future for you (hopelessness).
    1-Never 2-Sometimes 3-Often
20. Feeling that you can do nothing in life (helplessness).
    1-Never 2-Sometimes 3-Often
21. Feeling not worth living or want to do self-harm.
    1-Never 2-Sometimes 3-Often

IV. Physical self-assessment:

22. Lazy to do daily exercise.
    1-Never 2-Sometimes 3-Often
23. Increased dietary fat, calories intake.
    1-Never 2-Sometimes 3-Often
24. Substance abuse (narcotic drugs/smoking/alcohol).
    1-Never 2-Sometimes 3-Often
25. Takes stress even in routine activities.
    1-Never 2-Sometimes 3-Often
26. Finding fault in everything (self and others).
    1-Never 2-Sometimes 3-Often
27. History of hypertension/diabetes among parents.
    1-Never 2-Sometimes 3-Often
28. High risk sexual behavior (multiple sexual partners).
    1-Never 2-Sometimes 3-Often

V. Reproductive health section (girls only):

29. How frequent are your menstrual periods?
    1: 21–35 days 2: <21 days 3: >35 days
30. How is your menstrual flow usually?
    1: Normal 2: Very less 3: Clots
31. Lower abdominal pain during menses/mood changes.
    1: No/mild 2: Moderate 3: Severe
32. Burning sensation during urination.
    1: No 2: Sometimes 3: Always
33. Itching in the groin/vulva.
    1: No 2: Sometimes 3: Always
34. Vaginal discharge?
    1: Pearly white 2: Excess 3: Foul smell
35. Do you have any of these suggesting polycystic ovarian syndrome (PCOS)? *(obesity, acanthosis, hirsutism)*
    1: None 2: Hair growth 3: No menses

VI. Sexual self-awareness:

36. Do not feel uncomfortable discussing sex/sexuality.
    1-Often 2-Sometimes 3-Never
37. Readily accept sexuality-related changes within me.
    1-Often 2-Sometimes 3-Never
38. Positively conscious about how attractive I look.
    1-Often 2-Sometimes 3-Never
39. Can handle sexual thoughts and feelings.
    1-Often 2-Sometimes 3-Never
40. Self-stimulation/masturbation does happen.
    1-Often 2-Sometimes 3-Never
41. Firm believer of commitment in relationship.
    1-Often 2-Sometimes 3-Never
42. Aware of sexual orientation (homo-, hetero-, bisexual).
    1-Often 2-Sometimes 3-Never

VII. Spirituality self-awareness:

43. Believe in religious activities and experiences.
    1-Often 2- Sometimes 3-Never
44. Use religion and faith to face life problems.
    1-Often 2- Sometimes 3-Never
45. Believe that God has sent me here with a purpose.
    1-Often 2- Sometimes 3-Never
46. My religious belief has an impact on my behavior.
    1-Often 2- Sometimes 3-Never
47. Believe in prayers and religious practices.
    1-Often 2- Sometimes 3-Never
48. Have tolerance for other religions and their beliefs.
    1-Often 2- Sometimes 3-Never
49. Have firm belief in religious basic concepts. (such as the Creator of the world, concept of soul, life after death).
    1-Often 2- Sometimes 3-Never

VIII. Partner Assessment Scale Trivandrum (PAST)—(For married only)

(Note: How do you rate yourself in the following domains?)

50. *Reality:* With all the good and bad in marriage overall real-life rating.
    1: >50% 2: 25–50% 3: <25%.
51. *Fantasy:* Fit in with your own fantasy-partner/child/profession.
    1: >50% 2: 25–50% 3: <25%
52. *Support:* Financial support/family support/peer's support.
    1: >50% 2: 25–50% 3: <25%
53. *Attitude:* Whether taking the concept of marriage seriously.
    1: >50% 2: 25–50% 3: <25%
54. *Sexuality:* Sexual satisfaction with husband/wife-overall assessment.
    1: >50% 2: 25–50% 3: <25%.
55. *Personality:* Giving type (Enjoy by giving pleasure to partner).
    1: >50% 2: 25–50% 3: <25%.
56. *Value system:* Both partners share common values.
    1: >50% 2: 25–50% 3: <25%

SUGGESTED READING

1. Nair MKC, Russell PS, Mammen P, Abhiram Chandran R, Krishnan R, Nazeema S, et al. ADad 3: the epidemiology of anxiety disorders among adolescents in a rural community population in India. Indian J Pediatr. 2013;80 Suppl 2:S144-8.
2. Nair MKC, Shyamal Kumar, Aswathy LA, Meenai Z, Dalwai S, Ahmed S, et al. Self-counseling for mother of children with autism spectrum disorder. Indian Journal of Developmental and Behavioral Pediatrics. 2022;Inaugural Volume (1); 3-6.
3. Panda PK, Gupta J, Chowdhury SR, Kumar R, Meena AK, Madaan P, et al. Psychological and behavioral impact of lockdown and quarantine measures for COVID-19 pandemic on children, adolescents and caregivers: A systematic review and meta analysis. J Trop Pediatr. 2021; 67:fmaa122.
4. Russell PS, Nair MKC, Chandra A, Subramaniam VS, Bincymol K, George B, et al. ADad 9: Suicidal behavior in anxiety disorders among adolescents in a rural community population in India. Indian J Pediatr. 2013;80 Suppl 2:S175-80.
5. Russell PS, Nair MKC, Shankar SR, Tsheringla S, Jakati PK, Chembagam N, et al. ADad 7: Relationship between depression and anxiety disorders among adolescents in a rural community population in India. Indian J Pediatr. 2013;80 Suppl 2:S165-70.

3 SECTION

Case Discussions

26 CHAPTER

Grief Counseling

Neema Sitapara

INTRODUCTION

Grief includes a range of feelings from deep sadness to anger. The process of adaptation to loss is unique for each person depending on his/her background, beliefs, relationship to what was lost, and other factors. Grief is often seen as interfering with life, rather than being intrinsic to life. Children are often protected not only from death but also, from the little losses that happen throughout lives, leaving them with little experience to face them. An early, high level of distress is one of the predictors that the person is at risk for a poor bereavement outcome. In earlier times, much of grief resolution was supported and facilitated through religious organizations, families, rituals, and customs. More recently, with changes in many of these areas, more people struggle to process intense loss and turn to counseling. **Box 1** gives an understanding of terminologies associated with grief.

PHASES AND PSYCHOLOGICAL REACTIONS TO LOSS

A grieving individual passes through three main phases after loss:

1. *Acute or self-protective phase:* Initial shock, denial, and disbelief. The individual may feel dissociated from the world around. Sometimes, initially there is an intellectualized acceptance (e.g., "Well, he was suffering anyway").
2. *Confrontation:* This is the most intense experience of grief. Emotional extremes are common in this phase. Rapid and large swings in emotions like anxiety, anger, and guilt are felt which lessen over the time. Intermittent denial may also occur. The individual often confronts the family members or friends with questions of "What if....?" "Did I do enough?" "What did

BOX 1: Terminologies.

- *Grief:* The *experience* of losing someone to death (also includes other losses)
- *Mourning:* The *process* the bereaved passes through to adapt and become accustomed to the death or loss
- *Bereavement:* The *loss* the individual feels while they learn to adapt
- *Grief counseling:* Involves helping people facilitate uncomplicated, or normal, grief to a healthy adaptation within a reasonable time frame
- *Grief therapy:* Involves more specialized techniques associated with treating people with abnormal or complicated grief reactions (prolonged, delayed, and exaggerated)
- *Complicated grief*[*]*:* Grief experiences that do not seem to be normal—abnormal, atypical, unresolved, and difficult. It can be characterized by:
  - Delayed or absent grief
  - *Conflicted grief:* This is a distortion or prolongation of one of the phases of grief or one of the phase components. The most common are extreme anger or extreme guilt
  - *Chronic grief:* The grief is fresh all the time. This may be indicative of a very problematic relationship, relationship with a lot of unfinished business or with dependence
  - Psychiatric disturbances associated with grief, e.g., depression. This may delay the resolution of grief
  - Physical illness associated with grief

[*]Complicated grief can be identified using the Inventory of Complicated Grief (ICG-14, score ≥30 at least 6 months after the death). It is prevalent in about 10% of grieving individuals.

I do wrong?" "What did I do to deserve this?" "Why wasn't it me?" Sadness and despair, inability to concentrate or process information, and preoccupation with the deceased are common. Restlessness, lack of ability to initiate and maintain organized patterns of activity, difficulty completing or concentrating on tasks at work, and withdrawal from the very people who help are other social manifestations. Physiological or somatic manifestations of grief which bring the bereaved into physicians' offices may include anorexia and other gastrointestinal disturbances, loss of weight, sleep disturbances, fatigue, weakness, palpitations, shortness of breath, etc. Spiritual issues like the basic search for meaning in life, feeling of abandonment, and anger toward God/higher power may occur.

3. *Reestablishment:* Grief gradually softens to an acceptance of the reality with decline in symptoms. Periods of grief may resurface at specific times such as holidays and birthdays.

Popular psychological models of grief are given in **Table 1**. All aspects of an individual being are affected by grief. A sudden, unanticipated death causes more intense reactions. There is no particular sequence or timetable for processing grief. Daily life stressors will affect the journey of grief adaptation and reconciliation. One can never get over with the loss but can learn to live with the loss. Grieving is a journey and not a task to be accomplished. The survivor is often directionless for a time as the future plans with the deceased have suddenly collapsed, creating a void.

Parents should also be aware about a child's understanding of death and related issues to help a grieving child **(Table 2)**. The grieving process in children can be quite different and complicated as compared to adults as shown in **Box 2**. Identifying the warning signs and timely referral to specialists is the key to a better outcome in a grieving child.

TABLE 1: Popular models of grief.

Elisabeth Kübler-Ross	***J W Worden***
Five stages of grief model	Four tasks of mourning model
The five stages are: 1. Denial 2. Anger 3. Bargaining 4. Depression 5. Acceptance	*Four tasks are:* 1. To accept the reality of the loss 2. To work through the pain of grief 3. To adjust to life without the deceased 4. To maintain a connection to the deceased while moving on with life
The stages may differ in sequence or may be missed	*Subgoals of grief counseling aligned with each task are:* • Increasing the reality of loss • Helping deal with emotional and behavioral pain • Supporting in overcoming obstacles to readjustment • Helping maintain a bond with the deceased while feeling comfortable reinvesting in life

TABLE 2: Children's understanding about death.

Age	*Concept*	*Concerns*
0–3 years	• No clear concept about death • May sense grief in others	• Equate death with sleep if explanations comparing death to sleep were given earlier; may develop fear of sleep and night • May develop distress symptoms when protected from pain of grief
3–6 years	• Often consider death as a reversible event (images from cartoons show death is temporary) • They also may express magical thinking that they caused the death or that they can reverse the death	May regress and show disturbances in eating, sleeping, and toileting
6–9 years	Aware of the finality of death but do not believe it is universal	Can become aggressive or overly clingy as they grieve
By age 9 or 10 years	Most children understand that death is final and universal	Can participate in funeral and grieving process after preparing them ahead of time for what they are to see

BOX 2: Grief in children.

- Children of all ages grieve and their expression may be different than that of adults
- Their grief may be expressed through extremes of behavior—from being aggressive to being very passive
- They need to be educated about grief, funerals, and issues related to death in terms they can understand. Parents must involve themselves in this process
- They often appear to be participating normally in usual activities even while harboring strong feelings
- Although their grief appears brief and is expressed intermittently, parents and caregivers should be aware that it often lasts longer and requires constant support and monitoring
- Their grief processing changes with development and new understanding. Children re-experience and revisit their grief during significant life events

ATYPICAL GRIEF IN CHILDREN AND INDICATIONS FOR THERAPY OR REFERRAL

- Continued denial of the death
- Prolonged anger
- School problems that are not resolving
- Behavioral problems that did not exist before
- Persistent physical symptoms such as sleep disturbances and eating disorders
- Social withdrawal
- Disabling or persistent regression.

ROLE OF GRIEF COUNSELOR

Worden has given 10-step guidelines for grief counseling. They make the grief counseling process effective no matter what the circumstances of loss and grief were.

1. Help the bereaved actualize the loss. Questions like "When did it occur?" and "How was the funeral?" help the individual come to the reality of death.
2. Help the bereaved identify the wide range of reactions to trauma, such as numbness, frustration, guilt, confusion, anger, anxiety, sadness, and feelings of helplessness. This enables them to get a sense of relief and encourages them to start exploring options.
3. Assist living without the deceased while helping the bereaved identify the problems that arose since the loss.
4. Help to find meaning in the loss to create a feeling that the death of the loved one was not in vain.
5. Facilitate emotional relocation of the deceased and help the survivor realize that the lost person can never be replaced and that it is alright to form new relationships as a part of the process in moving on.
6. Provide time to grieve. To recognize critical times when pain resurfaces and assist the client to prepare in advance for them.
7. Interpret normal behavior of clients reassuring and acknowledging their emotional reactions as being natural, normal, and expected.
8. Allow for individual differences. Listen to the individual's concerns and expressions sensitively and caringly and help them grieve in their own unique ways.

9. Examine defenses and coping styles. Identify both functional and dysfunctional coping strategies and help clients explore more effective coping mechanisms.
10. Identify pathology and refer especially where there is complicated grief involved.

CASE VIGNETTE

Riya, 15 years old, lost her father and grandmother during the COVID pandemic in a short span of 2 months. Studying in 10th grade at that time, she was given mass promotion with the entire batch. After initial trauma and shock, she seemed to settle down in grade 11 and aspired to crack NEET to study medicine. Her mother, now the lone earning member of the family, took charge of the grocery shop owned by Riya's father. Riya's mother herself struggled to cope with her personal and financial crises. Riya started having headaches and difficulty in sleeping at night for 2 months. Whenever her mother tried to convince her to focus on studies and fulfill her father's dream, she got upset. She started deteriorating in academics and had frequent anger outbursts at home. Her headaches worsened. She was brought by her mother to the counselor seeking help for her behavioral issues.

After the initial rapport-building session, Riya could vent out her feelings of grief which had been bottled up mainly due to confusions and lack of self-awareness. She outwardly tried to be strong but could not resolve her grief. She believed sharing her sadness and stress with her mother would add to her burden. Riya felt lonely, anxious about future without her father, and struggled in her studies. She missed her grandmother and felt that God was punishing her.

Assessment

Depression was ruled out using Beck's Depression Questionnaire.

Setting Goals

Grief resolution, breakdown of disempowering beliefs, developing coping skills, and managing academic stress and anxiety were the goals set after discussion with Riya.

Parental Counseling

The mother was counseled and educated about grief, its impact on adolescent mind, and associated issues. She was advised to spare some special time with Riya remembering happy family moments spent in the past with father and grandmother.

- *Interventions:* Riya was helped by validating her feelings, increasing self-awareness by journaling, breaking her irrational beliefs, building up coping skills, and creating new routine with her mother. The following coping strategy was also discussed with Riya and her mother:
    - *Companioning:* Companioning is when a grief therapist acts as a companion who actively listens to the feelings of a grieving individual without analyzing or trying to fix things. The therapist simply provides a safe space to express emotions.
    - *Bibliotherapy:* Reading stories of loss, and how the bereaved worked through these emotions, can support an individual in his/her own healing journey. This technique can be especially helpful for those in rural communities with limited access to counseling or therapy.
    - Restoring routine can restore a sense of normalcy. Guiding to starting hobbies and projects can help one move forward while one continues to process the grief.
    - *Expressing emotions through art:* Drawing, painting, and writing are all common grief therapy techniques for adults and children.
    - *Preserving objects of connection:* These provide grieving people with a powerful continual bond with someone they have lost. Symbolic objects represent something about the lost person or situation like a birthday photo. Linking objects are items that evoke a sense of the lost person in the griever, such as parents holding on to their deceased child's stuffed animal. Objects of connection mostly serve a positive, adaptive function in the grieving process. Sometimes, they can be maladaptive.
- *Creating rituals:* Rituals help one channel his/her grief into a particular activity. Common grief rituals include lighting a

candle, visiting the grave, taking a daily walk, and preparing a favorite meal for the loved one. Rituals having significance both to the deceased and to the survivor are especially effective.

If the experience of loss and grief is unique, then counseling interventions that address those experiences must prioritize that uniqueness.

John Welshons, in his book "Awakening from Grief", states: "So there is no way to apply systems, rules or emotional road maps. Our job is to be a presence, rather than a savior. A companion, rather than a leader. A friend, rather than a teacher".

CONCLUSION

Bereavement and grief are a normal part of the human life. Grief is not an illness but a multidimensional, transformational and unique experience having physical, cognitive, behavioral, social, cultural, spiritual and philosophical foundations. Inadequately managed grief can cause dire consequences in children. Validation is the heart of grief counseling. Acceptance and explanation about grief is reassuring and supportive in itself.

SUGGESTED READING

1. Humphrey KM. Counseling strategies for loss and grief. Virginia: American Counseling Association; 2009.
2. Librach SL, Abrahams P. Ian Anderson Program in End-of-Life Care. Module 13. Grief and Bereavement: A Practical Approach. University of Toronto; 2004.
3. Keeran D. Loss and Grief Counseling Skills: The Practical Wording of Therapeutic Statements and Processes. California; 2010.
4. Wheeler-Roy S, Amyot BA. A Field Manual, Grief Counseling Resource Guide. New York: New York State Office of Mental Health, Bureau of Education and Workforce Development; 2016.
5. Worden W. Grief Counselling and Grief Therapy: A Handbook for the Mental Health Practitioner, 5th edition. New York, NY: Springer; 2018.

27 CHAPTER

Anxiety

Shubhada Khirwadkar

INTRODUCTION

Anxiety disorders are among the most common mental health conditions affecting adolescents, often presenting during a critical phase of emotional and psychological development. Adolescents may experience anxiety in response to academic pressures, social dynamics, identity formation, and life transitions. Understanding the clinical features, risk factors, and management of anxiety in this age group is essential for timely diagnosis and effective intervention.

CASE VIGNETTE

Ankita, a 16-year-old girl, was brought by her parents on the advice of her class teacher.

She had three episodes of fainting in her class in the past 2 months, twice during term examination and once a day before the Math unit test conducted last week.

The episodes were associated with giddiness, blackouts, tremors of both hands and feet, palpitation, sweating, and a feeling of extreme weakness. The fainting spells lasted for 5–7 minutes. She was awake and alert after she was made to lie down, her necktie loosened, and a few drops of water were sprinkled on her face.

SESSION 1

Rapport Building

After a brief introduction and greetings by the counselor, Ankita and her parents were welcomed with a smile. Detailed information about the fainting attacks was sought from the parents. (Prior information on fainting spells in school was already sought on the phone from the class teacher.) The parents were politely asked to wait outside when Ankita expressed her desire to talk alone.

Confidentiality about the conversation was expressed and its limits were summarized by the counselor. The conversation began with an open-ended question: "How can I help you, Ankita?" Gestures indicating counselor's interest in her story like forward bending, head nodding, congenial tone, eye contact, and a smiling demeanor were used while engaging her in a general talk about her school, friends, sports, films, books, and hobbies.

Ankita was initially hesitant but slowly started to talk about her irritability, restlessness, and being on the edge as examination approached. She was often unable to sleep, could not concentrate on studies and constantly worried about being unable to remember the studied portion, and went blank while solving paper, but was able to solve the same sums when she was back home. She refused to enter the examination hall for the class test citing fear of failing but appeared for it after much cajoling by her parents and encouragement by her teacher. This was followed by another fainting attack with sweating and palpitation. She also got tired easily and her headache while studying got relieved with some painkiller tablets.

There was no history of nausea, vomiting, absence attacks, aura, any other abnormal body movements, uprolling of eyeballs, falls, frothing at mouth, or loss of consciousness. There was no history of avoidance symptoms, obsessive thoughts, or repetitive behavior. There was no past history of seizure disorder, specific phobias, or separation anxiety disorder in childhood. There was no history of similar complaints in the family.

Complete systemic examination was done in the presence of a chaperone to rule out organic causes of fainting attacks like anemia, disorders of thyroid, high blood pressure, signs of adrenal pheochromocytoma, or any neurological deficit. No signs of raised intracranial tension were seen on fundoscopy.

HEEADSSS Interview

- *Home:* Ankita's was a nuclear family. She was an only child. Both parents were well-educated and successful professionals. High parental expectations about Ankita's academic achievements were often expressed by parents.

- *Eating:* Ankita had a balanced diet. There was no change in appetite. She was a vegetarian. She occasionally had junk food.
- *Education:* Ankita received average scores till IX standard. She always scored low in Math and also failed twice. She had special liking for music. She had won prizes in essay writing and liked to write poems in her diary.
- *Activity:* Ankita attended school and tuitions fairly regularly (6 hours of school and 4 hours of coaching classes). She was a good table tennis player and *attended music classes* but had stopped both now. She had very few friends. She liked to be alone in her room. She watched late night music videos on her own. She had no specific study or sleep schedule. She was concerned about putting on weight after her sports participation had stopped. She had great faith in Lord Krishna and visited temples regularly.
- *Drugs:* Ankita had never used psychotropic drugs but had twice been given low-dose alprazolam a few months ago, by her mother to induce sleep when she was unable to sleep after witnessing the the collapse and death of their neighbor. She had once indulged in hookah smoking at a party with friends.
- *Safety:* Ankita drove a nongeared two-wheeler, and wore a helmet while driving.
- *Sexuality:* She had been in a steady relationship with a classmate for the last 2 years. He supported her during stress of examination by giving her his notes. No sexual intimacy was revealed. Both families knew each other.
- *Suicide:* No thoughts of self-harm or suicidal attempts were reported.

On the basis of the counseling session, HEEADSSS, and systemic examination, a diagnosis of an anxiety disorder was considered and the following *investigations* were advised to rule out organic causes of anxiety:

- *Complete blood count:* Hemoglobin 12 g%; mildly hypochromic red blood cells (RBCs); rest within normal limits
- Triiodothyronine (T_3), thyroxine (T_4), and thyroid-stimulating hormone (TSH) levels within normal range
- Ultrasonography (USG) abdomen was normal (done to rule out adrenal medullary tumor).

SESSION 2

SCARED (Screen for Child Anxiety Related Disorders) tool for anxiety was used to obtain an objective assessment of anxiety and its severity and devise an appropriate framing of treatment. Ankita scored 30, which indicated severe anxiety. She also had a score of 8 on items specific for panic disorder with significant somatic symptoms (her fainting spells, intense sweating, and palpitation).

Differential Diagnosis of an Anxiety Disorder

According to Diagnostic and Statistical Manual of Mental Disorders, 5th edition (DSM-5), the major types of anxiety disorders are generalized anxiety disorder (GAD), panic disorder, social phobia (or social anxiety disorder), separation anxiety disorder, selective mutism, specific phobia, agoraphobia, and substance/medication-induced anxiety disorder.

Ankita's symptoms, psychological tests, and investigations pointed toward the diagnosis of a panic disorder, which often responds well to an eclectic approach to treatment.

- *GAD:* Although Ankita had difficulty in concentrating, irritability, and sleep issues which indicated a generalized heightened anxiety, there was no prolonged, vague, unexplained state of intense fear or hyperarousal affecting other areas of her life. Her distress was more specifically related to her exam schedules.
- *Obsessive-compulsive disorder (OCD):* Was ruled out because there was no history of obsessive, intrusive, and repetitive thoughts, actions, or rituals affecting her daily functioning
- *Panic disorder:* Unwarned, sudden, overwhelming, apparently senseless attacks of fear encompassing her entire being associated with sweating, shortness of breath, tremors, palpitation, and dizziness (autonomic overload) associated with her three fainting spells, all pointed toward a panic disorder. The apparent activating trigger was an approaching examination.
- *Post-traumatic stress disorder (PTSD):* Ankita did show an avoidance behavior in terms of avoiding to appear for her test out of extreme anxiety (fainting spells) and had sleep difficulties; PTSD was ruled out because there was no history of a traumatic event any time before the past 6 months and neither

hyperarousal and hypervigilance nor re-experiencing the horror of any traumatic event was present in her.

- *Social phobia (social anxiety disorder):* Ankita did not have any specific phobia and no fear of interacting with people.

With Ankita's typical symptoms and high score on items of panic disorder on SCARED, the final diagnosis as per DSM-5 was generalized anxiety with panic disorder.

Goals of Treatment

The presence of some features of generalized anxiety in Ankita which could be long standing and the need to deal with the issues of immediate concern warrant a clarity on short-term and long-term goals of treatment. The goals of treatment of an anxiety disorder can be well set if problems are clearly defined.

- *Cognitive issues:* Ankita's severe anxiety with somatization was closely linked to her extreme anxiety of failure to do well in school, especially in Math. During her first two counseling sessions and on HEEADSSS evaluation, the following faulty cognitions became evident:
  - She was an undeserving daughter of well-educated and academically successful parents.
  - She felt ashamed and guilty that her failure brought disrepute to the family name.
  - Inability to score well in Math put a stamp of "failure" on her entire personality.
  - Approaching Xth board exams the next year added to her academic burden.
  - She used avoidance measures rather than learning ways to handle her anxiety.
- *Long-term goal:* Incorrect, illogical cognitions to be corrected using the cognitive behavioral therapy (CBT), but such therapy needs a sizable number of sessions over a period of time. This is a long-term goal which can be achieved with 10–12 sessions on CBT.
- *Short-term goals of therapy were formulated partnering with Ankita:*
  - Learning relaxation techniques, meditation, visual imagery, drugs to reduce anxiety

- Reducing the frequency of panic attacks using systematic desensitization
- Learning study skills and time management
- Building confidence in problem solving in Math with one-to-one coaching
- Reassuring parents that these skills would equip her to tide over anxiety issues
- Taking teachers on board for sensitive and empathetic approach

Interventions

Generalized anxiety and panic disorder requires a flexible and patient approach as either many children are reluctant to take drugs or parents refuse to use drugs with a concern that drug therapy could be addictive. A counselor needs to explain the safety and usefulness of drugs along with the counseling sessions.

SESSION 3

Session 3 was utilized to discuss the plan of treatment with Ankita and asking her preference to work on the goals. Her parents also were explained about the nature and type of and time for therapy. She was keen to learn the fear-handling techniques first.

Drugs

Ankita was put on fluoxetine 40 mg once a day to reduce her generalized anxiety levels. She had some issues in waking up that settled in a couple of weeks. Antianxiety drugs are known to reduce the somatic symptoms perceptibly and calm down the patients well so that they become amenable to counseling and adhere to the homework and practice suggested by the counselor.

Therapy Plan

Further counseling sessions were planned on alternate days for the next 2 weeks.

Cognitive behavioral therapy sessions were also planned weekly for the next 10 weeks to help Ankita deal with her faulty thoughts and change them into reasonable ones.

Counseling Challenges

- *Permissions:* If systematic desensitization is to be carried out in school to reduce anxiety, support and participation of parents, school, and teachers in the plan is vital.
- Adherence issues and irregularity of scheduled sessions are often a challenge for the counselor as school assignments deadlines, exams, etc., take priority.

SESSIONS 4–6

Ankita was taught the progressive relaxation technique (PRT) which she needed to practice at home daily. In this, while lying down with eyes closed, successive muscle groups are made tense and then relaxed one after another along with "self-talk" of "getting relaxed". This was to be carried out before she went to bed daily and practice sessions were done in the clinic and the parents were asked to videograph the procedure at home and send it so that the counselor could suggest any corrections if needed.

SESSION 7

Deep breathing and practicing mindfulness meditation was also taught and daily log was kept of 5–10 minutes practice. Use of these relaxation techniques on identifying the cues of panic or gripping fear (rapid heart rate, sweating, light-headedness) was also taught.

SESSION 8

Study Skills

SQ3R (survey, question, read, recite, and review) technique, topic mapping, and use of memory cards were taught to build study skills. Homework of keeping a log of time spent on various activities was given.

The importance of a healthy diet, exercise, and adequate sleep was explained to her. She agreed to cut down her media use.

Daily coaching sessions on Math were discussed and started with her aunt who was asked to give feedback on Ankita's progress.

SESSION 9

Parental Counseling

In a follow-up session with parents, they were asked for feedback on her progress. The alternate-day schedule of her sessions was changed to weekly ones and clubbed with CBT sessions. They seemed relieved to see a reduction in Ankita's symptoms. They were counseled on supporting their daughter in healthy relaxation activities and agreed to restart her weekend music lessons and 1 hour of table tennis daily. They helped to coordinate with the school for organizing systematic desensitization sessions.

SESSION 10

Teachers were counseled regarding having a sensitive and empathic approach toward Ankita and their cooperation was sought in organizing school-based sessions. Their help was crucial in organizing these sessions.

Stepwise systematic desensitization to reduce the fear of entering the examination hall was done. In the first step, Ankita was taken to the adjacent corridor near the hall and asked to stand by the wall and practice deep, conscious breathing whenever thoughts of fear or panic occurred. Gradually, over a week, she could enter and then stay in the hall for 5 minutes with someone alongside. After a month, she could solve a few questions in the hall for 15 minutes. With the encouragement of schoolteachers, she finally appeared for her test after 3 months and received passing marks. The relaxation techniques and self-talk that Ankita learnt to use in stressful situations also helped her in participating in a school debate.

SESSIONS ON COGNITIVE BEHAVIORAL THERAPY, LIFE SKILLS

The sessions on cognitive restructuring continued weekly for 4 months. She was taught the technique of questioning her self-defeating thoughts and how critical and creative thinking skills can be used in handling problems. Some planned sessions were missed, which is a common feature with school-going adolescents getting busy with exams and assignments. Overall improvement in anxiety level was noted by Ankita herself, both parents, and teachers. Fluoxetine was gradually withdrawn over 2 weeks.

TERMINATION

The sessions were terminated after 8 months when no panic/fainting attacks were reported. No booster sessions could be conducted as her Xth board tuitions started.

CONCLUSION

Effective management of adolescent anxiety requires a holistic, multidisciplinary approach that includes psychoeducation, cognitive-behavioral strategies, family support, and, when necessary, pharmacological treatment. Early identification and intervention can significantly improve long-term outcomes, helping adolescents navigate challenges with resilience and fostering healthy emotional development.

SUGGESTED READING

1. Bandelow B, and Michaelis S. Epidemiology of anxiety disorders in the 21st century. Dialogues in Clinical Neuroscience. 2015:7(3);327-35.
2. Craske MG. et al. Anxiety disorders. Nature Reviews Disease Primers. 2017:3;17024.
3. DSM-5-TR (Diagnostic and Statistical Manual of Mental Disorders, 5th Edition, Text Revision)–Gold standard for diagnostic criteria.
4. Hofmann SG, Asnaani A, Vonk IJ, Sawyer AT, Fang A. The efficacy of cognitive behavioral therapy: A review of meta-analyses. Cognitive Therapy and Research. 2012:36(5);427-40.
5. Mayo Clinic–https://www.mayoclinic.org/diseases-conditions/anxiety/symptoms-causes/syc-20350961
6. National Institute for Mental Health (NIMH)–https://www.nimh.nih.gov/health/topics/anxiety-disorders

28 CHAPTER

Romantic Relationship

Newton Luiz

INTRODUCTION

Romantic relationships are a part of the emotional and social development of the adolescent. They are an opportunity to learn how to choose a trustworthy life partner, manage sexual feelings, negotiate conflict, communicate needs, and respond to a partner's needs.

CASE VIGNETTE

16-year-old Priya, an 11th-grade student, was brought by her mother to her regular pediatrician as she was underperforming in her studies for 6 months. Her mother had repeatedly caught her talking softly on the phone during study time and suspected that she was in a romantic relationship.

INITIAL ASSESSMENT

History: Priya admitted that she was unable to concentrate on studies for few months. While eliciting the history, Priya's mother started scolding her, accused her of being in a relationship, and blamed her boyfriend for a fall in academic performance. This embarrassed Priya, and she requested the pediatrician for a consultation session in private. The mother readily consented for a counseling session at the adolescent clinic, the next day.

Examination: General and systemic examinations were normal.

Impression: Adolescents with recent decline in academic performance in a probable romantic relationship

STEPS OF COUNSELING

1. *Building rapport:* The pediatrician greeted Priya and assured her that the discussion was confidential, and nothing would be revealed to her parents without her permission. His friendly demeanor and nonjudgmental attitude helped Priya to openly discuss sensitive issues during the HEEADSSS interview **(Table 1)**. She admitted that she was in a relationship with her school senior, Ravi, and needed help to sort out a few confusing issues.
2. *Assessment:*
   Priya said that she loved Ravi very much but was confused about personal boundaries and physical intimacy. The pediatrician said that it was a wonderful feeling to be in love and have a healthy mutually enhancing romantic relationship. It was normal for her to be confused about issues that were not in accordance with her personal value system. He reassured her regarding the availability of help and helped her to frame and prioritize goals for life.
3. *Goal setting:* Priya set the following goals for herself:
   a. *Short-term goals:*
      i. Resolve confusion regarding her relationship with Ravi
      ii. Improve academic performance
      iii. Re-strengthen relationship with parents
   b. *Long-term goals:*
      i. Lead a happy and healthy life with her parents, husband, and children
      ii. Become an English college professor

   The pediatrician outlined a plan of 10–12 fortnightly sessions for her. Priya agreed with this plan.
4. *Interventions:* The technique of motivational interviewing was used to counsel Priya by expressing empathy, developing discrepancy between current behavior and life goals, building self-efficacy, and at times rolling with resistance

   First session:
   a. *The pediatrician started by acknowledging Priya's admirable strengths:*
      i. Had the support of a very loving family

TABLE 1: HEEADSSS screening.

Home	Nuclear family. Had a good relationship with father, mother, and brother. Father was autocratic and a very strict disciplinarian. She felt that he would not like Ravi and feared getting scolded by him. Lately, her mother's taunts regarding her character were disturbing her. She did not want to reveal about Ravi to her parents
Education	Above average in studies until 5 months ago. Presently, she was barely able to pass exams. Was not finding enough time to study, had poor concentration, and lacked focus due to her deep involvement in the romantic relationship. Her teachers and school friends were unhappy with her performance. Her ambition was to become an English college professor
Eating	Liked eating nutritious homemade food. Occasionally ate fast food. Had no body image concerns
Activities	Played badminton for 30 minutes daily with Ravi and longer sessions on weekends. Spent 4–5 hours/day on the mobile talking to Ravi. Slept for 3–4 hours/day. Lately, her sleep was disturbed
Drugs	Disapproved of smoking and alcohol intake. Ravi drank alcohol with his friends, once or twice a week
Suicidality	Not depressed, just confused and distracted. No suicidality
Sexuality	• Regular monthly periods with normal flow • Was in a romantic relationship with Ravi since 5 months, he was very handsome and fun to be with, she felt uncomfortable and distressed when he forced her to hug and kiss him, he disturbed her during study hours by phoning frequently, he was cajoling her to accompany him for an overnight holiday with his friends next month when her parents and brother were to go for a pilgrimage. This was her first serious relationship. She had not had sexual intercourse with Ravi and said that she wanted to wait until marriage
Safety	Was scared of her father's anger bouts. He had never been physically abusive. Also feared Ravi's disapproval and anger when she refused physical intimacy and was apprehensive that he might break the relationship

   ii. Had a specific goal in view of becoming a college professor
   iii. Played badminton regularly, an enjoyable and energetic game
   iv. Had clear and well thought-out personal values, such as her respect for academics and career and her disapproval of alcohol, smoking, and premarital sex

b. *Priya was asked to list out the disturbing effects of the relationship on her life:*
   i. His persistent phoning at study time was seriously affecting her studies and might ruin her future study plans and job prospects.
   ii. It was jeopardizing her relationship with her parents, by causing her to hide the truth from them.
   iii. Time spent alone with him was exciting, yet stressful at times, due to his undue persistence for physical intimacy.

c. *Priya was then asked to list out features of a healthy romantic relationship:*
   i. Your beloved is very important to you but not the only priority in your life.
   ii. You love being with him, and you feel quietly contented even when he is not around.
   iii. You are faithful, have mutual respect, and trust each other. You do not emotionally blackmail each other or force each other to indulge in activities without consent, especially under the effect of alcohol.
   iv. You should have plenty of time for family and other friends, for study and sleep, for games and hobbies.
   v. You both have independent opinions on many issues, and you enjoy discussing them. You may agree to disagree at times.
   vi. You do not need to hide the relationship from family or friends.

The pediatrician closed the session by summarizing the key points discussed and giving her a homework assignment of analyzing her current relationship with Ravi and the changes that she aspired for.

Second session: In this session, Priya discussed the changes that she would like to see in her present relationship:

a. They should agree on a mutually suitable time for phoning or texting each other.
b. He should respect her need to study and not force her into physical intimacy.
c. They should spend more time just being together and getting to know each other.
d. He should stop drinking alcohol.

The pediatrician appreciated her for completing the assignment and for her clarity of thinking. He discussed basic negotiation skills and taught her how to say "no" effectively and assertively. He also discussed safe responsible sexual behavior, sexually transmitted infections, contraceptive use, pregnancy, abortion, healthy media use, sexting, flag signs of an abusive relationship, sexual abuse reporting strategies (to parents or pediatrician or police by calling 100 and/or Childline at 1098), legal age of consent under Protection of Children from Sexual Offences Act, and coping with a breakup. As homework, he asked her to discuss with Ravi the changes that she wanted in her relationship. He suggested that this discussion should preferably take place in a public place like a garden or shopping mall to ensure safety, lest he gets angry and violent.

FOLLOW-UP SESSIONS

In follow-up sessions, Priya revealed that using effective communication skills, she could easily convince Ravi for not going out for a holiday (due to impending exams) and had negotiated for a phone talk time of 1 hour/day. She expressed keenness to learn time management and study skills to improve academic performance. She was taught conflict resolution and interpersonal skills to improve her relationship with parents. After eight sessions, Priya expressed a desire to end the counseling sessions as her academic performance had improved and she was happy with her relationship with Ravi and her parents. She had introduced Ravi to her parents, and they had accepted him as her friend and asked her to maintain personal boundaries with him. The counselor started preparing her for the termination of counseling sessions.

TERMINATION

A week later, Priya requested for an "urgent" counseling session. At the session, she revealed calmly that a drunken Ravi had ditched her for another girl when Priya had refused to get sexually intimate with him. She said though she felt a little sad for losing him, she knew that it was the best thing that could have happened to her—for her health and mental well-being. She thanked the pediatrician for "preparing her in advance" for such an event. She said that she hoped to find a worthy life partner in the future and expressed a desire to focus exclusively on studies for now. The pediatrician appreciated her appropriate decision-making and coping skills. He reassured regarding his availability for further counseling sessions. Priya said that she felt confident about handling her issues and declined the offer. The pediatrician said that he respected her decision and asked her to continue with annual adolescent wellness visits. Priya agreed to do so.

PARENTAL COUNSELING

With Priya's assent, her parents were counseled over three sessions. They were encouraged to talk to Priya in a respectful and loving tone about morals, family and social values, peer pressure, risks of premarital sex, responsibility, the right to mutual respect and consent, breakups, and to set limits on sexual relationships and mobile use for chats or talks. They were asked to be role models of good relationships. They were further told that if a parent is violent or dominates over the other, the adolescent may conclude that it is the norm in any relationship. In the later sessions, they were appreciated for their efforts to get to know Ravi better and for accepting him as Priya's friend. They were also asked to discuss with Priya in a factual manner their dislikes, if any, about Ravi.

CONCLUSION

Adolescent romantic relationships need sensitive and careful management. Counselors should impart developmentally appropriate comprehensive sexuality education with an open and nonjudgmental attitude. Motivational interviewing is an effective technique for making healthy decisions. Parental/caretaker education and collaboration are vital while managing a sexuality-related issue in adolescence.

SUGGESTED READING

1. Avilés TG, Finn Christine, Neyer FJ. Patterns of Romantic Relationship Experiences and Psychosocial Adjustment From Adolescence to Young Adulthood. Journal of Youth and Adolescence. 2021;50:550-62.
2. Collins WA, Furman W, Welsh DP. Adolescent Romantic Relationships. Annu. Rev. Psychol. 2009;60:631-52.
3. Couture S, Vaillancourt-Morel M-P, Hébert M, Fernet M. Associations between Conflict Negotiation Strategies, Sexual Comfort, and Sexual Satisfaction in Adolescent Romantic Relationships. The Journal of Sex Research. 2023:60(3);305-14.
4. Giordano PC. Relationships in adolescence. Annual Review of Sociology. 2003;29:257-81.

29 CHAPTER

Problematic Screen Use

Neha John, Manoj Kumar Sharma, Nitin Anand, Rajesh Kumar

INTRODUCTION

Addiction refers to the chronic, relapsing, and compulsive act of engaging in specific behaviors despite associated negative consequences. Other than substance addiction, i.e., excessive use of psychoactive substances, excessive engagement in non-substance behaviors (e.g., gambling, eating, sex, etc.) can lead to behavioral addictions. One sub-category of behavioral addictions are so-called technology addictions including addictions to internet/screen use, online gaming, pornography, social media and so on. These addictions are seen often in the adolescent population due to the need for the internet and its ubiquity in their lives. However, data regarding the spread of these newly identified addictions is not very robust. One meta-analysis found prevalence of moderate and severe Problematic Internet Use (PIU) among Indian school going adolescents as 21.5% and 2.6%, respectively (Joseph et al., 2022).

Such addictions can negatively impact physical and mental health, academic performance and social functioning. Comorbid psychological and physical health problems usually have a bidirectional relationship. As with any other mental health disorder seen in children or adolescents, psychosocial factors are an important factor in the process of development and maintenance of an addiction. The COVID-19 pandemic and subsequent lockdown lead to a substantial increase in the use of screens and internet for a large number of adolescents. This seems to have triggered technology addiction in vulnerable children and adolescents. Due to the complex and interrelated nature of such factors, multiple areas need to be targeted for effective treatment. The following case vignette was chosen to illustrate some of these complexities.

CASE VIGNETTE

Mr VA is a 17-year-old male, studying in 12th grade, single, belonging to a family of upper-middle socioeconomic status. He was brought to a tertiary specialty clinic for management of technology addiction by his mother and presented with complaints of excessive screen use, disinterest in pleasurable activities, delayed sleep schedule, poor self-care, reduced interaction with family members, and school refusal for 3 years. According to his mother, excessive screen use began during the COVID-19 lockdown as it was required to attend online classes and was the only way to keep in touch with friends and classmates. In 2021, after school reopened, he regularly attended school but increased screen use continued. VA's academic performance in 10th grade was below his own expectations and his screen use further increased. He also changed schools and had difficulty forming a new peer group. During this time, he lost interest in most activities he engaged in and would use his phone throughout the night to watch YouTube videos or Instagram reels up to 10 hours continuously. Over time, VA refused to go to school or play with friends, claiming he was disinterested. According to VA's mother, he was academically above average with no history of any behavioral issues. Previously, he had been taken to a counselor but dropped out after three sessions. VA's household consisted of his parents and younger sister. His mother was a homemaker and father worked in the IT sector who frequently traveled for work. Mother is reportedly a worrier and emotionally closer to VA. She was under pharmacological and psychotherapeutic treatment for depression. Father is reportedly short-tempered, critical, uses alcohol excessively, and has a poor relationship with VA. There is a history of marital discord between both parents.

STEPS OF COUNSELING

Rapport Building

As is often the case with adolescents and especially those with problematic screen use, VA was reluctant to begin counseling and claimed he did not have any issues. He agreed to come to counseling at his mother's insistence. This coupled with previous experiences of counseling meant rapport building was especially crucial and prolonged. VA came across as intelligent and psychologically minded. He was easy to interact with and seemed to appreciate the opportunity to engage in unstructured, nonjudgmental, and attentive discussion with the counselor. Over time, the counselor was able to introduce ambivalence regarding his current behaviors vis-à-vis his values and goals in life, thus motivating him to engage in counseling.

Assessment

Once rapport had been established, a detailed clinical history was taken. It was established that problematic screen use was primarily a coping mechanism to avoid distressing emotions. He was assessed using the Internet Addiction Test (Young, 1998) and screen use was found to be in the category of problematic Internet use. It helped him avoid feelings of social isolation and inadequacy in academics as well as sports. It also allowed him to stay awake at night and sleep during the day, so he could avoid interacting with family members. It was also seen that there was significant guilt for his mother's distress as well as anger toward his father. It was revealed that VA used to consume alcohol sporadically when greatly distressed.

Goal Setting

The collaborative goals that were set in counseling were:

- Increase engagement in meaningful activities
- Manage emotions in a healthy manner
- Reduce time spent on screen use
- Communicate emotional needs and difficulties to parents and friends.

Psychoeducation and Interventions

Initially, VA was psychoeducated about his diagnosis and problematic screen use as a tool for avoidance. Intervention focused on the following:

- Engaging in pleasurable activities
- Value-based behavioral activation
- Facilitating experiential acceptance using mindfulness exercises
- Learning healthy coping skills

- Learning to communicate openly and assertively with family members
- Spending meaningful time with family members.

Termination

Termination was initiated once VA's mood and engagement in his activities significantly improved. He started going to school regularly and engaged in extracurricular activities. Feedback from parents indicated that he was engaged in family activities and willing to communicate. VA's screen use was in better control and he was able to prioritize other activities over it. Termination carried out over a few sessions focused on integrating the insights gained and skills learned through counseling. VA was appreciated for the significant changes he had made.

Parental/Caregiver Counseling

Throughout the counseling process the parents, primarily the mother, were additionally seen by the counselor. This was to psychoeducate them regarding VA's difficulties, engage them in providing an accepting environment to VA, supporting him as he did homework tasks from counselling, and update them on his progress. The close collaboration with the mother facilitated a speedier and holistic treatment.

REFERRAL INDICATIONS AND COLLABORATIONS WITH MULTIDISCIPLINARY HEALTH PROFESSIONALS

Once a detailed clinical history was taken from VA, it appeared he was suffering from a major depressive episode with a probable diagnosis of dysthymia. He was referred to the Child and Adolescent Psychiatry Department of a tertiary medical center where pharmacological management was initiated. Though indicated, couple therapy was deferred as VA's father was reluctant for the same. Instead, VA and his parents were referred to a private family therapist to address the significant issues in the family context that were contributing to VA's presentation, which would also help engage the father more in VA's treatment.

CONCLUSION

VA's case highlights a typical but complex presentation of problematic screen use, seen at a tertiary speciality clinic. With the widespread struggle faced by adolescents and families to manage technology use and the lack of specialized care, there is a dire need for all health professionals who come into contact with adolescents to play their part. Paediatricians often have trusted, long-term relationships with families that may last through years of development.

As most adolescents are not forthcoming with these difficulties and often don't recognize their screen use as problematic, the formation of a good alliance with the adolescent becomes the most important factor for successful intervention. Pediatricians should routinely inquire about/screen for problematic technology use. They may psychoeducate the adolescent and their family about the possible adverse consequences of excessive screen use. If the adolescent and family is amenable, they can advise simple lifestyle modifications, aimed at balancing online and offline lives of the whole family. Rather than attempting to cut down screen use directly, it may be easier to increase the amount of spent engaging in offline activities. They may also advise steps to improve family well-being and communication. In cases where such interventions don't seem to be effective, the adolescent has multiple comorbidities or the family functioning is significantly impaired, they should make a referral to a mental health professional. Ultimately, pediatricians can help prevent the development of these disorders through regular screening and early intervention as well as promotion of healthier screen use in families.

SUGGESTED READING

1. Joseph J, Varghese A, Vijay VR, Dhandapani M, Grover S, Sharma SK, et al. Problematic internet use among school-going adolescents in India: a systematic review and meta-analysis. Indian J Community Med. 2022;47:321-7.
2. Sharma MK, Anand N, Tadpatrikar A, Marimuthu P, Narayanan G. Effectiveness of multimodal psychotherapeutic intervention for internet gaming disorder. Psychiatry Res. 2022;314:114633.
3. Young KS. Caught in the Net: How to Recognize the Signs of Internet Addiction—and a Winning Strategy for Recovery. Hoboken, NJ: Wiley; 1998.

30 CHAPTER

Eating Disorders

Chitra Dinakar, Preeti M Galagali

INTRODUCTION

Eating disorders have varying clinical presentation and are best diagnosed by eliciting details pertaining to 'attitudes to eating' and measuring weight, height and BMI. All eating disorders are associated with an abnormal relationship with food and eating practices (food restriction or binging) with or without attempts at burning excessive calories. Body image concerns and comorbid mental health problems like depression and anxiety can coexist. Anorexia nervosa is a type of eating disorder that requires urgent referral to a trained adolescent psychiatrist.

CASE VIGNETTE

Fifteen-year-old Asha was brought for evaluation of extreme weight loss and excessive exercising over the past 6 months. She was originally 50 kg with a height of 150 cm and body mass index (BMI). She was doing well in school and studies in the 10th standard. However, over the past 3 months she has become withdrawn, avoids her favorite crafts class and meeting her friends, and prefers being alone in her room. Her exam grades have fallen and has difficulty sleeping. Her parents are very concerned about her dietary intake. She is unable to share the reason for her poor eating and gets angry with her parents when they force her to eat any kind of food, even her favorite dishes. She insists on eating alone and refuses to join her family for meals. She also locks her room door for prolonged periods and spends excessive time in the bathroom. She was always fond of skipping and continues to skip. However, her parents feel that she is also secretly skipping in the bathroom. She has also missed her periods for 4 months.

INITIAL IMPRESSION

Asha is likely to have depression with disordered eating, very likely an eating disorder such as anorexia nervosa (AN).

CASE DISCUSSION

Clues in the case that point to an eating disorder are that Asha gives no reason for food refusal, does not reveal about what is actually eaten and how much, gets angry when the topic of her poor food intake is brought up, and has behavior that indicates irrational attempts at burning calories (obsessive exercising) in secrecy. AN is a type of eating disorder where there is an extreme fear of gaining weight and a false perception of being fat in spite of being unacceptably thin. The adolescent could be very unhappy about their body image (weight and shape/size of body parts such as thighs, arms, and face). This disorder requires qualified psychiatry-guided pharmacotherapy and interventions along with counseling and can be associated with depression and/or anxiety. Asha needs to be referred to a physician and psychiatrist urgently after first-line counseling. The physician's role is to rule out other diseases with weight loss and to stabilize heart rate, blood pressure, organ functions, and metabolic abnormalities. Asha could take months to recover, averaging 3–6 months, and needs prolonged follow-up (2–5 years) even after recovery to prevent relapse.

STEPS OF COUNSELING (IN THIS CASE, FIRST CONTACT COUNSELING, PRIOR TO EARLY REFERRAL)

Rapport Building

Asha is likely resentful for being forced to see a counselor and is a difficult candidate for rapport building, which could take a full session. Here, the counselor started by greeting Asha and her parents and by introducing herself. On seeing the grimace on Asha's face, the counselor responded with an understanding smile and said that young people could sometimes be irritated when they are coerced for a counseling session and it is alright for her to feel the way she does. She further said to the parents, "I will spend some time with

Asha and you to understand the problem. I will try to help Asha find some relief from her difficulties. Maybe with your inputs (Asha's and parents') we can plan out the next steps". Asha and her parents agreed to an interview in private, and limits of confidentiality were explained to facilitate sharing without fear/stigma.

Assessment, Treatment, and Goal Setting

Severity

The counselor then assessed if Asha needed immediate referral to a physician by asking her and her parents for symptoms such as extreme fatigue, breathlessness, and fainting. This history was reported as negative.

Psychosocial History

A HEEADDSSS psychosocial history was elicited in private to identify "strengths" and priorities for goal setting based on Asha's identified priorities that align with improved health. Asha shared that her mother was too busy with housework and did not spend much time with her. This made her very sad. A priority goal was set to encourage shared time by reinforcing Asha's suggestion of having a meal and an evening walk with her mother. Asha also shared that she was concerned with her low exam score. She had missed many school days because of medical visits. A goal dear to Asha was to return to school at the earliest. The counselor suggested that her return to school was conditional to her complying with a minimum meal plan that would improve health and well-being and facilitate her return to school.

Feelings of Distress Linked to Food

Eating itself causes extreme distress in AN. There is a need to make a detailed daily diet contract (timing, number of meals, choice of food, quantity) and also involve the family for assisted implementation. Daily counseling is more effective in the initial days of treatment to ensure positive reinforcement for even apparent minor changes (minor changes from the family/doctor perspective, but achieved with major efforts from the adolescent's perspective). Only once a week weight check is done with an electronic scale, wearing the same dress, prebreakfast to minimize distress related to weight gain. The counselor needs to be prepared to handle the distress associated with gradual weight gain and set acceptable reasonable targets with the adolescent. Family-based therapy has the best outcome. Minor changes in diet proceed week on week balancing the distress associated with eating and the fear of gaining weight. Asha was gently guided toward an eating goal such as having a cup of *dal* with her rice/*roti* instead of plain *roti*. The meal plan accommodated her reasonable but not irrational or unhealthy choices related to food. The overall goal of counseling her was not just to gain weight or achieve a particular body shape but to develop and maintain a healthy relationship with food and overall health and well-being. Counselors need to understand the total diet approach in their management of the problem. The total diet approach suggests a variety of foods in moderation with no rigid restrictions on choices. The focus is on a sustainable healthy relationship with food and eating practices.

Asha required constant positive reinforcement for desired behavior and validation of her feelings of distress. The counselor used the technique of active listening to help her ventilate and share her difficulties and frustration with the situation. The counselor also focused on nonfood-related talk and activities that helped her shift her thoughts to other enjoyable activities such as craft, walk with mother, and reading a subject like social studies that she enjoyed, rather than indulging in vigorous physical activities.

Parental Counseling

Asha's parents were informed regarding normal adolescent health parameters and habits (not weight alone), mental well-being and parenting, strategies to handle a particular situation (like a tantrum from Asha when she is reminded of a particular contract she is breaking), and the need to collaborate with health professionals, and solutions were discussed regarding their disrupted routine because of their participation in her medical care, etc. It was emphasized that overprotection or permissive parenting of Asha can be detrimental. Problem-solving process was explained with examples. The need for family counseling was reiterated. A letter to the principal and class teacher was framed to explain school absences, the need for sensitive handling of academic deterioration, facilitating healthy peer relationships and involvement in extra academic activities such as craft work.

Referral and Collaboration

The parents were apprised regarding the need to collaborate with a multidisciplinary team of psychologist, nutritionist, psychiatric social worker, and adolescent health specialist. They were also informed about the requirement of prolonged follow-up for at least 2–5 years as the chances of a relapse were very high and to initiate transitioning to adult services by 16 years so that it could be completed by 18 years. By this time, Asha would be empowered to handle responsibly not only the medical problem but also adapt to changing demands of education and career choices while continuing treatment. Asha was explained about the referral to the multidisciplinary team. Both Asha and her parents agreed to the referral. Asha did well under the multidisciplinary team. Two years later, her BMI was normal, she was following a healthy lifestyle, was compliant with the prescribed antidepressant therapy and follow-ups, and had joined a fashion designing course where she was doing well academically.

CONCLUSION

Diagnosing eating disorders requires a high index of suspicion. They are complex to manage and require a dedicated team approach to address various interventions and follow-up. A systematic approach with a multidisciplinary team comprising Adolescent physician, Psychiatrist, Psychologist/Counsellor, Nutritionist and Social worker is conducive to long term recovery.

ACKNOWLEDGMENT

We thank the patients and parents who placed their trust in the treating team, Departments of Pediatrics and Psychiatry, Unit of Child and Adolescent Psychiatry, St. John's Medical College Hospital, Bengaluru, Karnataka.

SUGGESTED READING

1. Abraham A. Eating disorders in adolescents. Ind J Adolesc Med. 2019;1:11-4.
2. DSM-5-TR criteria for anorexia nervosa. [online] Available from https://dsm.psychiatryonline.org/doi/10.1176/appi.books.9780890425787.x10_Feeding_and_Eating_Disorders. [Last accessed September, 2024].
3. Jose JN, Dinakar C, Srinivasan R, Krishna S, Ahmed A, Joseph J. Anorexia nervosa: a missed diagnosis. Ind J Adolesc Med. 2019;1:33-5.
4. Kumar MM, Argo T, Chang J, Cifra N, Docter AD, Galagali PM, et al. Preventing nutritional disorders in adolescents by encouraging a healthy relationship with food. J Adolesc Health. 2020;67:875-9.
5. Vaidyanathan S, Menon V. Research on feeding and eating disorders in India: a narrative review. Indian J Psychiatry. 2024;66:9-25.

31 CHAPTER

Suicidal Behavior

Preeti M Galagali, Chitra Dinakar

INTRODUCTION

Suicide is a common cause of adolescent mortality in India. Most suicidal behavior in adolescence are impulsive. Causes of suicidal behavior are multi-factorial and include family problems, failed love relationships, poor academic performance, mental and chronic medical disorders, substance use, poor coping skills to life stressors and child abuse. Brief interventions, empathetic counseling and referral to psychiatrists is known to decrease recurrence of suicidal behavior and save lives.

CASE VIGNETTE

An anxious mother brought Rakesh, her 14-year-old son, for counseling when she noticed multiple parallel scars on his left forearm. A day earlier, Rakesh had revealed to her that the wounds were self-inflicted.

Initial impression: Nonsuicidal self-injury

STEPS OF COUNSELING

Rapport Building

The counselor, after the preliminary introductions, validated the feelings of distress and reassured Rakesh and his mother regarding the availability of help. The counselor requested consent from the mother and assent from Rakesh to talk with him in privacy. Rakesh and his mother agreed to do so.

Brief Risk Assessment

The limits of confidentiality were explained to Rakesh and a history was elicited regarding the forearm injury. He said that he had slashed his forearm with a blade 2 weeks ago in response to a "dare" by his peers. He confided that his classmates often ridiculed and teased him about his poor academic performance. He felt lonely and sad in the school and at home. When a group of classmates approached him to be a part of their group if he dared slashing his forearm, he readily did so. He further revealed that for 2 years, he had difficulty in completing the classwork and made many spelling mistakes but did well in oral exams. His teachers and parents were physically and emotionally abusive and often called him "lazy". He said that he aspired to become an Ayurvedic doctor like his parents. He was trained in yoga and had won many prizes at the national level. He was a Carnatic vocalist and had trained in music for 1 year. As his academic performance had dropped, his parents had stopped yoga training in the last 1 year. His parents showed favoritism toward his 10-year-old sister who was brilliant academically. She loved him very much. He said that he had suicidal ideas in the past; 6 months ago, when he felt distressed by poor performance in exams and parental abuse. He had never made any plans to commit suicide and had never made a suicidal attempt or nonsuicidal self-injury in the past. He said that for 2 months he had not experienced these thoughts as he had promised his sister to be her lifelong companion. The counselor appreciated the bonding and affection between the siblings, exceptional talent in yoga, and desire to become a doctor. The counselor expressed empathy by saying that at times, it becomes difficult to cope with distress and peer pressure and that "safe" coping, problem-solving, and assertive skills need to be learned and imbibed by everyone. Rakesh nodded in agreement with the counselor. The HEEADSSS assessment revealed risk and protective factors **(Box 1)**.

Rakesh was categorized as "low risk for suicide" as he had no current suicidal thoughts or plans.

Interventions

Ventilation

To facilitate ventilation, Rakesh was asked details about his relationship with parents and asked about the good times, if any, that they had spent together as a family. Rakesh admitted that most of the time, he shared a warm relationship with his parents but his

BOX 1: Risk and protective factors.

Risk factors:
- Poor academic performance (suspected learning disability)
- Abuse by teachers and parents
- Negative peer pressure
- Suicidal ideation in the past

Protective factors:
- Yoga
- *Ambition:* Ayurvedic doctor
- Strong sibling bonding
- *Hobbies:* Carnatic vocalist

academic performance triggered conflicts. His younger sister often helped him to complete notes. He enjoyed the family outings to the neighborhood park during holidays. His classmates often ignored him in school. Apart from his class teacher who was very kind and supportive, all the other teachers reprimanded him in public every day for the incomplete school work. He was very distressed about his poor academic performance. The counselor recounted the supportive people in his life and sought his permission to speak about the issue of academic performance, bullying at school, and past suicidal ideation with his parents and teachers. Rakesh agreed to do so.

Formulating a Safety Plan

The counselor further said that as his well-being was of paramount importance, it would be preferable to formulate a safety plan along with his parents **(Box 2)**. The counselor also explained in detail the need to consult a psychiatrist and psychologist in the next few days to rule out mental and neurodevelopmental disorders and facilitate psychoeducational assessment and plan for academic improvement and mental wellness. Rakesh hesitatingly consented. He wanted the counselor to convey the same to the parents.

Parental Support, Lethal Means Counseling, Referral, and Collaboration

After revealing to parents the reasons for Rakesh's mental distress, their feelings of agony were validated and hope was instilled

BOX 2: Safety plan for Rakesh.

1. I get stressed by:
    a. Thoughts of not being loved by parents, teachers, and peers
    b. Not doing well in exams
2. Things that I can do to cope/distract myself:
    a. Yoga
    b. Singing
    c. Going for a walk in the park
3. I can call/talk to the following people, when in distress:
    a. Parents
    b. Sister
    c. Class teacher
    d. Counselor
4. Telephone helpline: 1098

    Reminder: I am precious. My life is precious. One thing that makes life worth living is my desire to be a lifelong companion to my sister and to become an Ayurvedic doctor.

    Signatures: Rakesh Mother Father Counselor

that self-harm and suicides are preventable. They were given psychoeducation regarding impulsive behavior and emotional reactivity in adolescence. They were counseled to:

- Remain calm, supportive, and reassure Rakesh regarding help with academic issues
- Discuss and sign the safety plan
- Fix an appointment with the psychiatrist and psychologist for a psychoeducational assessment in the next few days to assess the severity of the learning disability, remedial education, and board accommodations, if required
- Nurture Rakesh's self-esteem by spending quality time with him, communicating effectively, appreciating his strengths of yoga, singing and of being a lovable brother, and consider restarting yoga training
- Build positive parenting skills, nurture both children with equal love and affection and avoid favoritism
- Facilitate life skills training for Rakesh with focus on assertive, problem-solving, and coping skills

- Remove Rakesh's access to sharp objects at home
- Discuss with the class teacher regarding ways to ensure personal safety at school, antibullying policy, and support in academic issues.

Follow-up

The counselor collaborated with the psychiatrist, psychologist, parents, class teacher, and sibling to follow up Rakesh's mental well-being over the next few months. After 3 months, Rakesh's academic performance had improved, he had a few friends in school, he was undergoing regular remedial education and dialectical behavior therapy sessions, his relationship with parents and teachers was better, and he had won many prizes in yoga competitions. There were no further episodes of self-harm. Rakesh continued to follow up with the counselor once in 3 months for a year.

CONCLUSION

Adolescents are highly emotionally reactive and vulnerable to self-harm. All cases of self-harm should be referred to a psychiatrist after brief risk assessment and first-level counseling to instill hope and reinforce strengths. It is important to formulate a safety plan and provide caregiver support and lethal means for counseling. Multidisciplinary collaboration and regular follow-up of cases of adolescent suicidal behavior is essential.

SUGGESTED READING

1. Galagali PM, Aroor AR. Management of adolescent suicidal behaviour in office practice. In: Pemde H, Ratna Kumari TL, Galagali PM, Velmurugan (Eds). Adolescent Friendly Pediatric Practice. New Delhi: Jaypee Brothers Medical Publishers; 2024. pp. 256-67.
2. Galagali PM, Dinakar C, Bala P, Shah D, Gupta P, Rao C, et al. Indian Academy of Pediatrics Consensus Guidelines on prevention and management of suicidal behavior in adolescents. Indian Pediatr. 2022;59:553-62.
3. Galagali PM, Ghate S, Sai Prasad KVS. Teen Depression and Suicide Prevention. IAP Standard Treatment Guidelines 2022. New Delhi: Jaypee Brothers Medical Publishers; 2023. pp. 911-19.

32 CHAPTER

Strength-based Counseling: Practical Application

Sreyoshi Ghosh

INTRODUCTION

Strengths-based counseling is a therapeutic framework that focuses on a person's inherent strengths, resources, and resilience rather than their problems, weaknesses, or deficits. It is rooted in the idea that everyone has strengths and inner resources that can be harnessed to overcome challenges and promote personal growth. The following case vignette illustrates this approach.

CASE VIGNETTE

Master Anil is a 14-year-old boy who came with the chief concerns of feeling intensely anxious when having to go to school, resulting in school refusal. Previous consultations with healthcare providers had led to an excessive focus on making him return to school at any cost, with a host of behavioral interventions having been advised without much success. When Anil had not been able to comply with treatment recommendations, he had felt a deep sense of failure and shame and not wanted to go back to the treating clinician.

The initial evaluation suggested that he has social anxiety. Family dynamics such as parental and sibling anxiety were contributing to the maintenance of the problem, and appropriate feedback was given. Sessions focused on building awareness regarding the factors that contributed to Anil's anxiety surrounding going to school. It became evident that his aversion to school is rooted in deeply traumatic childhood incidents involving the school that are still difficult to revisit and process. He is a sensitive boy with trait behavioral inhibition and low sensory threshold, which has made it hard for him to feel comfortable in social situations. A prolonged period of social isolation during COVID made it doubly hard for him to return to school, and perceived rejection by one of his peers after school return contributed to his feelings of shame and inadequacy. Anil has high internalized parental and societal expectations which make it very hard for him to deal with perceived failures. Thus, the very fact that he experiences anxiety has been a source of marked distress, and he goes to great lengths to mask/suppress his difficult emotions, which tends to maintain them over a period of time.

Anil's strengths are that he is extremely bright, diligent, and perseverant in addition to being reflective and introspective. He has maintained strong relationships with his family members and has the interpersonal skills to ask them for help when he requires it. Despite experiencing considerable anxiety in the therapy room, he persisted in his efforts to understand himself better and work on himself.

It was decided that as he is able to study well in environments that he found safe and nonthreatening, thus changing his board from Central Board of Secondary Education (CBSE) to National Institute of Open Schooling (NIOS) so as to allow him to continue his education. He is good at chess, so he would go for classes that would allow him some opportunities to socialize with other children of his own age. At times when he would feel overwhelmed and want to discontinue, he would be encouraged to focus on the times when he had experienced some measure of success while interacting with others in his chess class. He would be encouraged to ask his family members for help when he encountered difficulties while studying or experienced distressing emotions, as strong family relationships were identified as an asset for him. Sessions with parents and joint sessions with parents and Anil were also conducted to further strengthen their attachment.

Therapeutic work also focused on helping him understand the impact of his difficult and traumatic life experiences on his current functioning and rigid beliefs about himself and the world that may have originated as a result of them.

Medication management consisted of low-dose (20 mg) fluoxetine, which helped in reduction of his anxiety.

FOLLOW-UP

With continued support and encouragement from his family and treating team, Anil completed his 10th board exams through NIOS and then rejoined regular schooling from 11th standard. His journey is a good example of how a child's return to normalcy can be facilitated by a focus on their abilities and strengths, rather than on focusing only on their deficits and attempting to correct them.

CONCLUSION

In the above case example, it is evident that a traditional behaviorist approach to school refusal which would focus solely on school return may not be appropriate for some children with high anxiety and past traumatic experiences and may even be damaging. An approach that is strengths based will empower the child and facilitate healing and recovery.

SUGGESTED READING

1. Buckingham M, Clifton DO. Now, Discover your Strengths. New York: Free Press; 2001.
2. Epstein MH. The behavioral and emotional rating scale: a strength-based approach to assessment. Diagnostique. 2000;25(3):249-56.
3. Frankl VE. Man's Search for Meaning: An Introduction to Logotherapy. New York: Washington Square Press; 1963.
4. Schlechter AD, O'Brien KH, Stewart C. The positive assessment: a model for integrating well-being and strengths-based approaches into the child and adolescent psychiatry clinical evaluation. Child Adolesc Psychiatr Clin N Am. 2019;28(2):157-69.
5. Selekman MD. Solution-Focused Therapy with Children: Harnessing Family Strengths for Systemic Change. New York: Guilford Press; 1997.
6. Seligman ME, Steen TA, Park N, Peterson C. Positive psychology progress: empirical validation of interventions. Am Psychol. 2005;60(5): 410-21.
7. Smith EJ. The strength-based counseling model. Couns Psychol. 2006;34(1):13-79.
8. Strong T, Pyle NR. Constructing a conversational "miracle": examining the "miracle question" as it is used in therapeutic dialogue. J Constr Psychol. 2009;22(4):328-53.
9. White M, Epston D. Narrative Means to Therapeutic Ends. New York: WW Norton; 1990.

Index

Page numbers followed by *b* refer to box, *f* refer to figure, and *t* refer to table.

D

Q

R

S

T

U

V

W

Y

Z